Dangerous Grains

Dangerous Grains

WHY GLUTEN CEREAL GRAINS MAY BE HAZARDOUS TO YOUR HEALTH

James Braly, M.D.
and Ron Hoggan, M.A.

AVERY
a member of Penguin Putnam Inc.
New York

Most Avery books are available at special quantity discounts for bulk purchase for sales promotions, premiums, fund-raising, and educational needs. Special books or book excerpts also can be created to fit specific needs. For details, write Putnam Special Markets, 375 Hudson Street, New York, NY 10014.

a member of
Penguin Group (USA) Inc
375 Hudson Street
New York, NY 10014
www.penguin.com

Library of Congress Cataloging-in-Publication Data

Braly, James.
Dangerous grains : why gluten cereal grains may be hazardous to your health /
James Braly and Ron Hoggan.
p.   cm.
Includes index.
ISBN 1-58333-129-8 (alk. paper)
1. Celiac disease—Popular works.   2. Gluten—Health aspects—Popular works.
I. Hoggan, Ron.   II. Title.
RC862.C44B73   2002   2002022748
616.3'99—dc21

Printed in the United States of America
20 19 18 17

Book design by Amanda Dewey

The ideas that shaped this book have come from myriad sources. Thanking the few identified here ensures overlooking the many others who have contributed their insights and perspectives, and we apologize in advance for these oversights caused by space limitations. Among the many people who contributed, Don Wiss, Jonathan Wright, Bob Machon, Ashton Embry, Anthony Marini, Garth Benson, and Michael N. Marsh stand out. Thanks also go to our families; to Betty Hoggan, who contributed her enduring support and the faith needed to persevere, and to Zack and Rachel Braly, for their loving support and inspiration.

Thanks should also be directed to the thousands of dedicated gluten and celiac researchers around the world who have educated and validated us in our journey of discoveries. In addition, very special thanks must posthumously go to Dr. Theron Randolph, renowned and beloved food allergy–clinical ecology pioneer and clinician, who intellectually grabbed hold over twenty years ago and has yet to let go.

Finally, we are grateful to the many individuals who generously allowed us to include their case histories as representative of our growing understanding.

CONTENTS

Are Wheat and Other Grains Making You Ill?

Religious tradition calls it the "Staff of Life." Most of us eat it every day. It's even a phrase from a well-known prayer: "Give us this day our daily bread." But a growing and undeniable body of research (reviewed in this book by my friend and colleague James Braly, M.D., and Ron Hoggan, M.A.) tells us that our daily bread (more specifically, wheat and related cereal grains) may be negatively affecting as many as 90 million Americans and may be a basic cause of illness for up to 10 million.

How can this be? Haven't we been told, over and over and over again, that grains, particularly whole grains, are a fundamental part of a healthy diet and should be eaten every day? Isn't this belief a part of today's "Gospel of Good Nutrition"?

It's undeniable that whole grains are good nutrition for some of us. But it's even more fundamental that there is absolutely no food that is good for everyone. Who hasn't heard or read the observation made thousands of years ago: "One man's meat is another man's poison"?

It's been known for years that certain whole grains (wheat, rye, barley, spelt, triticale, kamut, and possibly oat) are the cause of celiac disease. This intestinal-tract disease can vary from mild (gas, bloating, loose stools) to life threatening (malabsorption, weight loss, malnutrition) and is preventable/treatable by completely eliminating all of the aforementioned grains from the diet. But isn't celiac disease rare? Less than one in one hundred Americans are diagnosed with this problem. Why should the rest of us worry?

Over the last two to three decades, at an accelerating pace, researchers have demonstrated that the offending proteins in these cereal grains (including gluten, gliadin, and glutenins) can cause symptoms, and sometimes entire diseases, in nearly any area of the body, *and not involve the intestinal tract at all!* These problems are often called "non-celiac gluten-sensitivity symptoms and diseases," "gluten-sensitivity symptoms and diseases," or simply "gluten sensitivity." This last term includes, but is not limited to, celiac disease. It also includes problems caused by sensitivity to grain subfraction proteins such as gliadin and glutenins.

The scope of the problem is much greater than imagined even a decade ago. A list of more than one hundred and fifty diseases and symptoms associated with sensitivity to gluten and other grain proteins, compiled by prominent researchers, can be found in appendix D of this book.

I first became aware of the wide reach of gluten sensitivity in the 1980s when I read *Relatively Speaking*, a book first published in Australia and republished in the United States as *Your Family Tree Connection* (unfortunately this classic, basic reading for any health-care practitioner or serious student of health, is now out of print. It can still be found through online sources of used books). Written by Dr. Christopher Reading and Ross Meillon, it describes Dr. Reading's detective work in unraveling the causes of "undiagnosable" symptoms through close examination of family health history.

When in Australia in the late 1980s, I had occasion to visit Dr. Reading's office in a suburb of Sydney. On one wall was a chart that would be amazing to any health-care practitioner even today: a list of over one hundred individuals who had initially consulted Dr. Reading about what they assumed to be lupus (systemic lupus erythematosus, SLE). When they first saw Dr. Reading, all had had symptoms (fever, joint pains, and skin rash are among the most common) and positive blood tests. But since consulting him, everyone on the list had been symptom free with negative blood tests for five years or more! That's right: over one hundred people *cured* of lupus in the 1980s. Even in the United States of 2002, any lupus specialist will tell us that's impossible and resume writing prescriptions for Prednisone, a dangerous, synthetic version of the natural cortisone molecule.

How did Dr. Reading do it? His program included *complete elimination* of all grains from the diet, except rice and corn (it also included elimination of milk and dairy products combined with heavy nutritional supplementation both orally and intravenously).

On returning to the United States, I headed for the university medical library, where I found a short but very intriguing article in the British medical journal *Lancet*. The author pointed out that many autoimmune diseases shared a common genetic marker called "HLA-B8," much more commonly than would be expected by chance. The list of HLA-B8 linked diseases were as follows:

Addison's disease	Lupus erythematosus
Autoimmune hemolytic anemia	(systemic)
Celiac disease	Myasthenia gravis
Childhood asthma	Pernicious anemia
Chronic autoimmune hepatitis	Polymyalgia rheumatica
Dermatitis herpetiformis	Scleroderma
Diabetes mellitus	Sjögren-Larsson syndrome
Graves' disease	Thyrotoxicosis
Insulin-dependent diabetes	Ulcerative colitis
(type 1)	Vitiligo

The author's key point was that every one of these diseases except celiac disease is autoimmune—diseases thought to be caused by an internal "reaction against self." But celiac disease was known to be caused by an external agent, gluten (which includes gliadin and glutenins as well). The author asked: Could this external agent, gluten sensitivity, also be involved in causing the rest of these HLA-B8–linked diseases?

I thought Dr. Reading had proved this to be the cause in systemic lupus erythematosus (SLE) by helping over one hundred people to cure their "lupus" by (among other things) totally eliminating all gluten-containing grains from their diets. So, since the 1980s, every time anyone consults me for any of these conditions, I recommend absolute avoidance of all gluten-containing grains (I also recommend absolute avoidance of milk and dairy, comprehensive allergy testing and desensitization, gastric analysis, large quantities of omega-3 essential fatty acids, many oral and intravenous vitamin and mineral supplementations, and testing and treatment with DHEA and testosterone. A complete explanation isn't possible here.)

The results have been fantastic (compared to "conventional treatment," which usually consists of Prednisone prescriptions and other immune-system-destroying patent medicines). Although not everyone has been cured of these HLA-B8–linked diseases, a very high percentage of them have had major improvement or complete remission. The exception has been established type 1 diabetes, where already-destroyed islet cells cannot be brought back to life, even by a gluten-free diet, and insulin treatment needs to be continued. But without permanent gluten-grain elimination, the rest of the program won't work nearly as well for any of these problems.

This book has reminded me that gluten sensitivity not only extends far beyond celiac disease and the HLA-B8–linked autoimmune diseases listed above. Dr. Braly and Mr. Hoggan estimate that 90 million Americans may have non-celiac gluten sensitivity. They write that undiagnosed sensitivity to gluten, gliadin, and other grain proteins is

> the root cause of many cancers, autoimmune diseases, neurological diseases, chronic pain syndromes, psychiatric and other brain disorders, and premature death. There is also a clear causal connection with some cases of osteoporosis, epilepsy, learning disorders,

attention deficit disorders, infertility, miscarriage, premature births, chronic liver disease, and short stature.

They also include complete lists of other gluten sensitivity–linked symptoms and diseases. Although written well for any of us to read, this book carefully includes 383 citations for health-care professionals and serious students.

Dr. Braly is a longtime clinical investigator into allergy, sensitivity, and health. He emphasizes that anyone who has gluten sensitivity also has other food sensitivities, and frequently many of them. I completely agree with his view that gluten/gliadin/glutenin sensitivities (along with milk/dairy sensitivity) are often "basic" or "root" sensitivities, which then lead to the development of many other allergies and sensitivities. When gluten sensitivity (or milk/dairy sensitivity) is found, comprehensive allergy testing should always be done. But even though desensitization techniques can successfully eliminate other allergies and sensitivities, no one should try to desensitize gluten/gliadin/glutenin sensitivities in order to stay well. They should be permanently eliminated from the diet of anyone who has a sensitivity to them.

Remember, gluten sensitivity includes but is not limited to celiac disease. While the "gold standard" for measuring celiac disease was an intestinal tissue biopsy, followed by gauging any characteristic changes in the biopsied tissue, many gluten sensitivity–linked symptoms and diseases listed in *Dangerous Grains* are *not* accompanied by changes in the intestine. Unfortunately, medicine as conventionally practiced doesn't accept this research-documented fact yet, even though it was first found to be the case by conventional practitioners years ago in the disease "dermatitis herpetiformis" (another HLA-B8–linked disease). Even though intestinal biopsies are often normal in dermatitis herpetiformis sufferers, the problem always clears up completely with strict gluten-grain elimination.

Fortunately, the development of highly accurate blood tests for gluten sensitivity has made diagnosis much easier and has greatly facilitated research. Before briefly mentioning the blood tests (which are detailed much better in the pages that follow), remember that Dr. Chris Reading figured out many of the disease and symptom connections with gluten sensitivity by examining family trees for various symptoms and diseases. Armed with a copy of *Dangerous Grains* for a comprehensive list of illnesses and symptoms, we can then do our own family trees of medical history and make an educated guess about whether we are at risk for a gluten-sensitivity problem.

The most sensitive and specific blood test for gluten/gliadin sensitivity presently available is the "tissue transglutaminase" (tTG). It's the test I've used since it became available in 1999. Others include "endomysial antibodies" (EMA), which check mostly "short-lived" antibodies, and "antigliadin antibodies" (AGA), which check "longer-lived" IgG antibodies as well as IgA antibodies.

Very important: We don't have antibodies to anything unless we've been exposed to it! If you've been avoiding all "gluten grains," the test will be negative even if you're truly gluten sensitive.

WHY SHOULD GRAINS BE SUCH A PROBLEM?

As previously noted, bread made from grains has been called the "Staff of Life." But research shows that agriculture and grain farming have existed at most for ten to fifteen thousand years, and humanity has been on this planet for much longer than that. For over 2 million years, our remote hunter-gatherer ancestors ate absolutely no grains at all! Agriculture and grain-eating have been around for ½ percent or less of the history of humanity, and many of us still haven't adapted to grains, especially gluten-containing grains (corn and rice cause their own set of problems).

This isn't "just a theory." Archeologists and other researchers have found that gluten-grain eating originated in the Middle East (Mesopotamia) and spread westward to the Mediterranean basin and northward into Europe. Since gluten sensitivity can cause or contribute to infertility, recurrent spontaneous miscarriage, amenorrhea (no menstrual periods), and low birth weight, there should be less surviving individuals with the HLA-B8 genetic characteristic in the areas first (and therefore longest) exposed to gluten-gliadin grains. This is, in fact, the case: The highest percentage of individuals who still have HLA-B8 (and other gluten sensitivity) genetic markers is found in the areas of Europe furthest away from the original source of gluten grains.

If we remain ignorant of the gluten grain–human genetic misfit (remember, this misfit doesn't occur in all of us, just a large percentage), it'll still be much longer than another ten thousand years before consumption of gluten grains removes all of us sensitive to them from the gene pool. In the meantime, there'll be a lot more illnesses, suffering, and premature death than we need to have, even given present knowledge.

If you have any suspicion that gluten grains may be contributing to your symptoms or illness, *read the rest of this book!* Then check with a health-care practitioner skilled and knowledgeable in both nutritional medicine and allergies. Such a practitioner is very like to be a member of the American College for Advancement in Medicine (ACAM, 1-800-532-3688, www.acam.org), the American Academy of Environmental Medicine (AAEM, 1-316-684-5500, www.aaem.com), or the American Association of Naturopathic Physicians (AANP, www.naturopathic.org). However, make sure to take a copy of this book with you to loan to the doctor (unless the doctor is Dr. Braly) because he or she will likely learn a lot from it, as I did.

If you find you have a symptom or disease related to gluten sensitivity, and you feel better after eliminating gluten-containing grains from your diet (along with other food allergies and sensitivities), give a copy of this book to a relative. Remember, Dr. Reading "figured it all out" without intestinal biopsies or blood tests, just by a careful examination of family trees.

Your Family Tree Connection first brought the public useful information about the health hazards (for many of us) of gluten-containing grains. *In Dangerous Grains*, James Braly and Ron Hoggan have given us a very much needed, and expanded, and updated picture of the health problems associated with gluten-containing grains—health problems affecting so many, but known by so few.

Jonathan V. Wright, M.D.
Medical Director, Tahoma Clinic
Kent, Washington

Author:
   Why Stomach Acid Is Good for You (2001, with Lane Lenard, Ph.D.)
   Maximize Your Vitality and Potency (1999, with Lane Lenard, Ph.D.)
   The Patient's Book of Natural Therapy (1999, with Alan R. Gaby, M.D.)
   Natural Hormone Replacement for Women Over 45 (1997, with John Morgenthaler)
   Nutrition & Healing Newsletter (1-800-851-7100, www.tahoma-clinic.com)

Our personal backgrounds and family histories provide powerful evidence of the hazards of eating gluten, as well as for the subtlety and variability of its devastating impact on human health. Our research was motivated by our own journeys along the path to wellness and by the health problems experienced by members of our families.

RON HOGGAN, M.A.

For years I was unaware of the cause of my discomfort. I just assumed that others were just as uncomfortable. I had variously been called emotional, picky, fussy, attention seeking, and a hypochondriac. I was diagnosed with an ulcer, a colicky appendix, and irreversible neurological damage related to a partial hearing loss. I also had a long history of chronic back and leg pain, which I attributed to injuries and aging. I accepted my hand tremors and chronic heartburn as reflections of my nervous nature.

All of those difficulties reached a low point on a December morning in 1994 when I was diagnosed with celiac disease. A fiber-optic tube, called an endoscope, was inserted in my mouth, down my throat, through my stomach, and into the upper part of my small intestine. With this device, tissue samples were taken to look for cancer. Thankfully, there was no evidence of malignancy. While the doctor would have to wait for a pathologist's report to confirm his suspicions, he was fairly confident that I had celiac disease and that I should begin to follow a strict gluten-free diet for the rest of my life.

By eliminating wheat, rye, oats, and barley from my diet, my world became a better place. More than seven years later, I now feel whole and healthy. Chronic pain from a knee injury of more than a decade before my diagnosis gradually faded away. Untreated, my celiac disease apparently interfered with its healing. Prior to diagnosis, I sometimes needed a cane to get around. Now the cane is collecting dust in the cellar. My vision and hearing improved. I experience fewer headaches and less back pain. The frequency and severity of acid indigestion are reduced. I no longer feel cold all the time.

After eliminating gluten grains, I realized how uncomfortable and chronically ill I had been for most of my life. My newfound wellness began my search for the tools to maintain and further improve my health. I have learned that such multiple, chronic medical conditions that often do not respond to conventional treatments are characteristic of gluten-sensitive and food-allergic individuals.

As a part of my journey to wellness, I underwent testing for common food allergies at the laboratory where Dr. Braly, my co-author, was medical director. The procedure, called IgG ELISA blood testing, led to further limitations on my diet. Although these restrictions were quite difficult in the beginning, I now consider myself very fortunate—most people with celiac disease are never diagnosed.

Despite considerable research indicating a frightening cancer risk among those with untreated celiac disease, and recent reports indicating that close to 1 percent of the apparently healthy U.S. population is affected by this disease, it is often considered rare and somewhat trivial by most of today's health professionals. Such perceptions are dangerously out of touch with the professional literature. I believe that my brother paid for these outdated beliefs with his life. I was to learn that all first-degree family members are also at high risk for this potentially fatal, genetically driven disease. As soon as I was diagnosed with it, my brother, mother, and children should have been invited for testing.

Sadly, this was not done. Instead, about ten months after my diagnosis, my brother, Jack, was diagnosed with non-Hodgkin's lymphoma. The largest, and what was presumed to be the primary tumor, was located near his kidney.

Despite considerable negotiation, including my brother's and my repeated requests, the attending physicians resisted testing for celiac disease on the basis that the tumor was not in the intestine and that his lymphoma was the first concern. No diagnostic testing was ever conducted. My brother died on November 18, 1996. His lymphoma may have been the result of untreated celiac disease. If so, he might have recovered, as other patients have, with a combination of conventional cancer treatments and an appropriate diet. Because of the general ignorance of celiac disease and its role in many types of lymphoma, my brother did not pursue a gluten-free diet to aid his battle against cancer. He was foolishly and incorrectly told that the diet is nutritionally inadequate and would compromise his chances of recovery.

My Daughter

When Kyra was twenty-four she visited the same specialist that diagnosed my celiac disease. He conducted an endoscopy to take tissue samples from her intestinal wall. The pathologist, another specialist who examines such biopsies under a microscope, noted a thickening of the bowel wall. Despite a large volume of research indicating that such a thickening is consistent with, and usually indicative of, celiac disease, that diagnosis was ruled out because more dramatic damage was not found.

A second opinion led to a diagnosis of celiac disease, but not before Kyra had suffered many more months of depression, lethargy, and abdominal pain.

Later, she wrote a feature article about her struggles, which appeared in the Summer 1998 issue of *Sully's Living Without*, a magazine devoted to people with food and chemical sensitivities.

JAMES BRALY, M.D.

As a child I suffered terribly from cow's milk–induced migraine headaches. Since dramatically reducing milk in my diet, I've not had a single migraine in over forty years. As an adult, when I overindulge in cheese, my joints and lower back begin to ache. No milk products, no aches or pain.

Years ago, while training for marathons, I would begin the day with a hearty breakfast that included a cup of regular coffee and whole-wheat or rye toast. I followed breakfast with a five- to ten-mile run. Almost invariably, when I ate bread with my coffee and then exercised vigorously, I would break out with extremely itchy hives on my upper back, chest, neck, face, and scalp, agonizingly lasting for one to two hours. I soon discovered that it was the gluten in wheat or rye that triggered the exercise-induced hives.

Today, if I eat breakfast and drink coffee, but without gluten-containing wheat or rye bread, no hives occur with exercise. Although not a celiac yet, I do have a definite gluten sensitivity, which expresses itself when I exercise. In addition, if I cheat by eating gluten-rich breads, pancakes, waffles, or bagels, with or without exercise, my abdomen will often swell almost immediately. I find myself secretly loosening my belt by one to two inches in order to breathe. Not surprisingly, without the gluten there is no bloating. Finally, I've noticed over the years that when overeating gluten cereals I will invariably experience a nagging, productive cough that vanishes predictably within a day or two on a gluten-free diet.

My son, Zack

From three to six years of age, Zack would complain frequently of deep, severe bone and muscle pain just above one or both knees, lasting for hours. The pain was often disturbing enough to prevent him from going to sleep at night. I can recall his mother and me spending many hours rubbing his legs in an attempt to give him some relief. I was reassured by his pediatrician that it was merely "growing pains," and he would grow out of it. Along with the leg pain, like I did as a child, Zack suffered from frequent, one-sided migraine-like headaches.

Zack was also a very short, small child the first six years of his life: his height and weight were always in the lowest 10th percentile for his age group. I suspected that something in his diet was stunting his growth and intuitively knew that he would not grow out of it until we changed his diet.

When wheat and other gluten cereals were eliminated from his diet, the leg pains dramatically vanished and have not returned (unless he cheats with spaghetti); he began growing rapidly. Within the first two months on a strict gluten-free diet he grew an astounding two inches. Today his height and weight fall in the upper 50 percent of his age group. His headaches occur rarely, if at all. Also, his food-induced headaches and leg pains are now a thing of the past.

So it is our personal experiences, combined with the struggles of our loved ones, that have led us into areas of research that we would not otherwise have considered. We now find that this research aided us both in providing sound advice on nutrition and testing to readers who are concerned about their health, and the impact of the modern Western diet.

We have discovered insights that would not have been possible if we had continued with the pro-gluten bias that was part of our education. Our research taught us great respect for Dr. Willem K. Dicke, Dr. Theron Randolph, and Dr. Curtis Dohan, whose heroic works have provided a foundation for understanding the health hazards of wheat. We have also been privileged to observe the encyclopedic memories of Dr. Loren Cordain and Dr. Michael N. Marsh, who have bridged the gap between theories and practical applications, clearing the path to human wellness. Their work has helped medical science leap forward in its understanding of celiac disease and a variety of autoimmune diseases, with special emphasis on the relationship between gluten, the immune system, insulin-dependent diabetes, and autoimmune thyroid disease.

Our research has also revealed the source of many, perhaps most, modern cases of osteoporosis, osteomalacia, and other bone diseases. Over 70 percent of untreated celiacs suffer from thinning of the bones. We have learned how those who suffer from a variety of highly prevalent gastrointestinal diseases such as canker sores, cancers, irritable bowel syndrome, Crohn's disease, ulcerative colitis, and esophageal reflux, often benefit from a gluten-free diet.

Our journeys of discovery have now become a joint quest to sound our warning about the dangers of a gluten-rich diet. We hope you will continue to listen.

Dangerous Grains

By beginning to read this book, you are taking an important step toward learning to control your health and well-being. Your journey of discovery begins before human civilization, beyond the origins of human farms and cities some ten thousand years ago. We take you back to look at prehuman primates. As the exploration progresses, we introduce you to cutting-edge research dealing with the dietary evidence found in the bones and teeth of our upright walking hominid ancestors who roamed the earth more than 2.5 million years ago. We highlight the convergence between modern medical research and archaeology that provides a basis for many of the insights we offer here. Frankly, we continue to be amazed by what we have learned.

We hope that you will use this knowledge as a springboard to dramatically improve your health and at the same time reduce your risk of developing many of the ailments caused or worsened by eating certain gluten grains.

Over 600 million metric tons of gluten-rich wheat are grown and eaten annually, making it the world's most consumed grain, well ahead of rice and corn. Yet it is also the grain, along with its gluten cousins, rye and barley, that puts tens of millions of humans at risk of premature death and gluten-induced illnesses such as autoimmune diseases, cancers, and osteoporosis. The dangerous impact of gluten not only bears up health issues here in the United States and Canada but also has profound morbidity and mortality implications for much of the world's wheat-addicted populations.

In those people who are genetically predisposed to gluten sensitivity, eating these grains has serious detrimental effects on the body's immune system. Gluten grains often trigger autoimmune diseases, such as insulin-dependent diabetes and hypothyroidism, where the immune system, instead of protecting the body, aggressively turns against it, causing chronic, potentially life-threatening diseases. In addition, gluten grains and dairy products contain morphine-like substances that affect behavior, cause learning difficulties, change emotions and moods, and cause or worsen neurological diseases. These food-derived drugs even alter how our immune system works and, as a consequence, dramatically increase our risk of developing many different kinds of cancer.

At the end of this book we provide detailed scientific references segregated by chapters so that if you choose, you can confirm our findings in recent, carefully scrutinized scientific and medical literature. We have also drawn information from our own clinical and personal experiences, including real-life reports from ordinary people who have experienced many of the symptoms and ailments caused by eating gluten grains, which, until very recently, have been thought to be universally healthful.

WHAT IS GLUTEN, AND HOW DOES IT CAUSE DISEASE?

Certain grains frequently eaten by humans can cause our immune systems to pathologically react to specific proteins. These disease-causing proteins are universally found within the seeds or grains of wheat, rye, barley, spelt, kamut, and triticale. The proteins are loosely called "gluten," and the cereal grains containing this gluten protein are collectively called the "gluten grains."

Gluten is made up of several subfractions or families of proteins. The scientific name for the most studied of these subfractions is "gliadin." Gliadin is found in all gluten cereals except for oats. Curiously and tragically, gliadin frequently causes the immune system to react as if it is not a component of nourishing food, but an invading bug or microbe or, worse, as though it is indistinguishable from normal organ tissues found in our bodies. These effects of gluten on the immune system, along with profound nutritional deficiencies that so often accompany gluten sensitivity, contribute to many modern diseases, which we will be exploring in this book.

Today, these abnormal immune reactions can easily be identified by appropriate laboratory and clinical testing. The test results can be used to help identify your risk of developing full-blown gluten-related diseases. Testing also identifies causal connections between diseases, symptoms, and gluten consumption; disease prevention and reversal often follow from a strict gluten-free diet.

WHAT IS CELIAC DISEASE?

Although medical researchers have known for well over fifty years that wheat and its near relatives cause celiac disease, most are still working toward a more complete understanding of this fascinating ailment.

Celiac disease, sometimes referred to as celiac sprue, is a genetically influenced condition that results from eating gluten. More specifically, celiac disease is an ailment whereby the inside lining of the small intestine, called the intestinal mucosa, is chronically damaged by gluten proteins and their interaction with the immune system.

As recently as 1990 in Europe, and 1996 in the United States, celiac disease was erroneously considered quite rare. On this side of the Atlantic, it was thought to affect about 1 in 4,850 Americans and Canadians. Thanks to innovative new laboratory testing, we now know that celiac disease was, and continues to be, grossly underestimated. More than 2 million Americans and Canadians suffer from this gluten-induced illness. This is approximately forty times the prevalence we were told less than a decade ago.

When actively sought, celiac disease is found in 1 in every 111 apparently healthy, symptom-free American adults, making it more than twice as common as cystic fibrosis, Crohn's disease, and ulcerative colitis combined.

The discovery that celiac disease cannot arise in a person who does not consume gluten grains was resisted vigorously for a number of years. The hesitation was likely because this information ran contrary to the widespread belief that these grains were a healthy food, especially in their whole-grain forms. The claim that they could cause widespread disease just didn't make sense. It was not until gluten was objectively shown to injure intestinal tissues, and a gluten-free diet consistently reversed this damage, that the discovery was finally, if reluctantly, accepted. That reluctance, as you will soon see, slowed recognition of the many ailments that can result from untreated celiac disease.

Undiagnosed celiac disease is the root cause of many cancers, autoimmune diseases, neurological diseases, chronic pain syndromes, psychiatric and other brain disorders, and premature death. There is also a clear causal connection with some cases of osteoporosis, epilepsy, attention deficit disorders and other learning disorders, infertility, miscarriage, premature births, chronic liver disease, and short stature. When a person is placed on a strict gluten-free diet, reversal of these conditions frequently occurs.

Despite these terrible consequences and the promise of cures, only one of every forty American celiacs is ever diagnosed and treated. The current rate of underdiagnosis is partly the result of the confusing, "atypical" array of signs and symptoms and, often, a complete absence of symptoms in the earlier stages of this disease.

WHAT IS NON-CELIAC GLUTEN SENSITIVITY?

Celiac disease is just one subset of gluten sensitivity, a message you will hear repeated throughout this book.

It is our considered opinion that whenever an individual's immune system is mounting an abnormal reaction to gluten, with or without symptoms, there is gluten sensitivity. Remember that gluten grains, along with dairy products, are the most common foods in our diet. If your immune system is identifying and abnormally reacting to any of the proteins found in gluten, this food poses a potential threat to your health.

Research into human genes now reveals that non-celiac gluten sensitivity, or immune reactions to gluten, may affect as many as 90 million Americans. The evidence suggests that these gluten-sensitive individuals face many of the same hazards associated with untreated celiac disease. They, too, have likely never suspected the underlying cause of their disease or how easily it could be prevented, halted, and often reversed. Gluten sensitivity is much more common, yet it is sought and diagnosed even less frequently than celiac disease.

The net result of this alarming rate of undiagnosed celiac disease and gluten sensitivity is a large population that is chronically ill, unresponsive to conventional therapies, and often desperately jumping from one doctor to another without relief.

To further confound the issue, untreated celiacs suffer a greater risk of infectious disease, and some evidence suggests a similar dynamic in non-celiac gluten sensitivity. Hence, even where antibiotics provide symptom relief, there may be an underlying, silent case of celiac disease or non-celiac gluten sensitivity that is increasing susceptibility to opportunistic infections. An excellent example of this dynamic is recurring middle-ear disease in children and infants, many of whom are gluten and dairy sensitive. More antibiotics are prescribed to treat the fever and pain, but the fundamental cause, food sensitivity, is never addressed.

The popular media and conventional nutritional wisdom, including the medical profession's traditional approach to nutrition, have created and continue to perpetuate this problem through inadequate, outdated dietary counseling. Attempts to universalize dietary therapies so that one-diet-fits-all influences the flawed claims against meats and fats, thereby encouraging overconsumption of grains.

Government-sponsored guides to healthy eating, such as the USDA's food pyramid, which advocates six to eleven servings of grains daily for everyone, lag far behind current research and continue to preach dangerously old-fashioned ideas. Because the USDA's function is largely the promotion of agriculture and agricultural products, there is a clear conflict of interest inherent in any USDA claim of healthful benefits arising from any agricultural product. Popular beliefs and politically motivated promotion, not science, continue to dictate dietary recommendations, leading to debilitating and deadly diseases that are wholly or partly preventable.

CELIACS TODAY SHOW DIFFERENT SYMPTOMS

To further confound this highly controversial political issue, authorities are reporting a fundamental shift in the presenting symptoms of celiac disease. Previously, it was a universal truth that all celiacs present in predictable ways with weight loss, muscle wasting, failure to thrive, chronic diarrhea, smelly stools, abdominal bloating and cramping, and perhaps iron-deficiency anemia. Today's celiac displays quite different symptoms, such as psychological depression, intestinal cancer, insulin-dependent diabetes, osteoporosis, short stature, canker sores, and/or chronic liver disease of unknown cause, to name just a few. In fact, well over 150 medical conditions have now been reported as overrepresented among gluten-sensitive individuals. (See appendix D for an extensive list of these conditions.)

A misconception also exists that celiacs are undernourished or emaciated. Yet, more of today's untreated celiacs are reported to be overweight or obese rather than underweight or wasted. The same research shows that the majority of untreated celiacs are well within the normal weight range. Contrary to prior beliefs, many research papers are reporting that most untreated celiacs have no abdominal symptoms at all.

Whatever health problems concern you, whether for a loved one or yourself, the answer is often found in diet and how the body reacts to foods. And the culprit may be the grain products you are eating and enjoying every day. The very food that provided the foundation of today's civilization, the food that is enshrined in the holy scriptures of several of the world's oldest religions, the food that is touted as the "staff of life," is really an unexpectedly common, serious threat to human wellness and existence. Yet even in industrialized countries, these grains serve as humanity's bulwark against starvation.

This is the extremely complex problem we face. Many people eat grains daily because they are cheap and abundant, yet science is reporting that these very same grains are bringing us to the brink of an enormous health crisis.

It is doubtful that the earliest farmers ten thousand years ago were aware of the health implications of the shift to gluten grains as a dietary staple. Even with today's sophisticated medical laboratory technologies and protocols, the health hazards of gluten-containing grains are being recognized by only a handful of medical researchers. This is due to absent or nonspecific symptoms early in the disease process and human bias rooted in history and psychology, accompanied by a universal reluctance to embrace radically new information. Acceptance of new ideas is often coupled with recognition of having been fundamentally wrong all along— a difficult admission for anyone.

MALADAPTATION TO A SILENT, DEADLY DISEASE

One may reasonably ask: If the symptoms of non-celiac gluten sensitivity and celiac disease can be absent, nonspecific, or minor well into adulthood, why is gluten considered a serious health threat to the gluten sensitive? Hans Selye, the father of stress research, answered that question very well in 1936. His discovery and description of the general adaptation syndrome, following his experiments with animals, offer a clear explanation of this dynamic.

Today, people adapt to eating gluten at a very early age. When first exposed to small amounts of gluten in cookies, crackers, soups, etc., some infants will become ill. If short lived, a gluten-induced illness is likely to be dismissed as one of the many normal cases of sniffles, colic, or diarrhea that occurs often during infancy. The connection between illness and eating gluten is rarely made, and infants, as a consequence, will continue to be fed a certain amount of gluten on most days. What is confusing is that they soon give the appearance of full recovery. However, if their illness was caused by gluten, they have only temporarily recovered from the symptoms but not from the cause of those symptoms—gluten sensitization. They have simply adapted, or maladapted, to this chronic source of dietary stress. Regular, frequent consumption of gluten, which is standard dietary practice in most households, maintains and perpetuates this maladaptation. The term used to describe this dynamic of adaptation to stress is "tolerance."

It is by means of such a tolerance that many gluten-sensitive individuals, despite their apparent state of good health, will develop a host of problems that appears to spring from nowhere. Some will develop short stature, bed-wetting, sleep disorders, headaches, or chronic fatigue, often accompanied by anemia. Others will suffer chronically from a vague unwellness, usually without a specific diagnosis, and rarely respond to conventional medical therapies. Still others will develop one or more autoimmune diseases, such as thyroiditis, chronic liver disease, or insulin-dependent diabetes. A small minority will suffer from deadly diseases, to which they appear to have little normal resistance and die at an early age. The majority of gluten-sensitive individuals will present a picture of apparently good to excellent health until the fateful arrival of an initial, often chronic illness. The sufferer will rarely, if ever, be aware of the underlying cause of this ailment.

Undiagnosed and untreated, many gluten-sensitive individuals continue to fall by the wayside as their diet depletes their nutritional status and immune systems, paving the way for the illness that besets them. Although it would be better to catch this insidious problem in infancy where it originates, it can be amazingly helpful to catch and treat this dietary condition at almost any age or stage of the disease. Even patients with advanced stages of cancer and AIDS are reported to improve when consuming a gluten-free diet.

An Australian psychiatrist, Dr. Chris Reading, has published accounts of a number of cancer patients battling clinical depression, which he treated with a gluten-free diet. The diet, in conjunction with conventional cancer treatments, resulted in a full recovery from the cancers in five out of six patients. Although this publication was not subjected to the scrutiny of the peer review process, the results are certainly consistent with that literature and our perspective.

SLOW ACCEPTANCE AND IMPLEMENTATION OF NEW KNOWLEDGE

Not only is the publication and dissemination of new knowledge painfully slow, most health professionals are slow to adopt new ideas from current research. This results in lengthy delays in the application of research to treatment, with patients suffering needlessly and dying prematurely in the interim.

There are a number of reasons for this unfortunate situation. Medical practitioners are often so overworked that many of them simply do not have the time to keep up to date on major medical breakthroughs. Even when doctors can devote some part of their busy days to studying current literature, it is literally impossible for one to keep up with the tens of thousands of international articles published monthly. For example, there are between ten and twenty thousand medical journals and newsletters published annually. The busy doctor must therefore prioritize which articles he will study. Predictably, most journals and reports will be set aside and never read. Studies dealing with the health hazards of grains will almost always be among those that are ignored. Many will see such articles as highly specialized, esoteric, and impractical. Physicians' prior training, often a decade or two behind the times, will have created the bias that gluten sensitivity is a trivial, rare aberration. Following the old adage "common diseases occur most commonly," most practitioners will choose to devote their time to studies and diseases that they believe are more likely to benefit a greater number of their patients. Hence, gluten sensitivity and celiac disease have been disregarded as irrelevant.

How This Book Can Help You and Your Doctor

We realize that most busy physicians will be unable to take time to look at yet "another health book" brought to them by a patient who might be considered one of the "worried well" or "grasping at straws." Here are some suggestions to help you overcome this potential problem. First, find the sections of this book that are pertinent to your own medical conditions, including those dealing with laboratory and clinical diagnosis. Next, to help your doctor gain confidence that the book's contents and your requests are science-based, look up the relevant citations at the back of the book under each chapter's list of sources. From that list choose several key articles, preferably with the most recent publication dates. Go to your local library with the list of sources and order or retrieve and photocopy the complete articles. When you have all the articles in hand, take them along when you visit your doctor. This science-based approach should increase the likelihood of your physician's confidence and cooperation for several reasons:

1. It will be obvious that you have already invested considerable time in exploring your health concerns and suspicions.

2. Because of their training, medical doctors are familiar with the rigors of the peer review publication process. Your doctor is much more likely to value this kind of literature.

3. If only because of issues of liability, your doctor will be less likely to dismiss researchers from many different medical centers around the world, reporting on carefully controlled experiments and data analysis.

With the peer-reviewed literature in your hand, you should feel comfortable asking your doctor to order the relevant laboratory testing identified in this book. With a little extra time and effort you can place yourself back in charge of your own health.

Persistent but out-of-date definitions of celiac disease formulated from the limited understanding of many years ago also contribute to a delayed acceptance of new information. Verified technical advances should lead to rapid redefinition, but too often they do not. For example, celiac disease was first described in 1888 by Dr. Samuel Gee, and reiterated by Dr. R. A. Gibbons. Their century-old view that celiac disease is solely a disease of malabsorption persists today. In 1888, celiac patients were identified by a failure to thrive and pale-colored, smelly, floating stools. Such stools, often in association with diarrhea, indicate a high-fat content, so these children were correctly perceived as malabsorbing dietary fat. Their description of the disease was limited to their understanding.

More recent advances clearly show poor absorption of essential vitamins and minerals among untreated celiacs, along with many other signs and symptoms throughout the body. However, the persistent notion of malabsorption in celiac disease has been overgeneralized and overemphasized, suggesting a general failure to absorb nutrients as the sole or primary defect. This conception of celiac disease is probably a defensible understanding of very advanced cases, but it ignores the majority who are either of normal weight or sometimes obese. Carbohydrate absorption often continues fairly normally.

As a consequence, an out-of-date definition has retarded research into celiac disease for over a century.

INTESTINAL BIOPSY AND REDEFINITION

The next step toward a better understanding of celiac disease resulted from Dr. Dicke's discovery in the 1930s that a wheat-free diet resulted in a full remission of symptoms. However, the acceptance of this radical discovery was slow, not garnering much attention until around 1950, when a surgical device was developed to biopsy tiny tissue samples from the small intestinal lining. It was this invention that belatedly led to redefining celiac disease during the 1960s. Thirty years after Dicke's discovery and eighty years after Dr. Gee's observations, celiac disease was still being considered a disease of malabsorption, but it was redefined to exclude other non-gluten diseases that cause fatty stools and failure to thrive. The new definition required intestinal damage, verified by a biopsy, which improves after excluding gluten.

This new definition relied on taking multiple intestinal biopsies on at least two separate occasions. These tiny tissue biopsy samples revealed a characteristic damage to the intestinal lining in patients with celiac disease. If the second biopsy, taken months later after beginning a gluten-free diet, showed that this intestinal damage decreased or disappeared, a confident diagnosis of celiac disease was made. The many other symptoms and signs of celiac disease were also dramatically reduced or eliminated by a gluten-free diet, of course, but curiously this has received less attention. Even now, the primary focus is on the intestinal biopsy and the resulting malabsorption.

Absorption of nutrients, especially fats and fat-soluble vitamins, is compromised by the simple reduction of absorptive surfaces in a damaged intestinal lining. As a consequence, malabsorption has continued to be identified as the primary feature of celiac disease; this is often thought to explain most, if not all, of its symptoms and signs. Again, this incomplete perception has led to the erroneous conclusion that patients with celiac disease must, by definition, be skinny, pale, overtly undernourished, and with a plethora of abdominal symptoms. This unfortunate bias places many patients at unnecessary risk.

NEW LAB TESTS, NEW DEFINITIONS, NEW HOPE

During the intervening period of sixty-five years since Dicke's discovery and fifty years since the development of tools to collect tissue specimens, huge strides have been made in almost every area of celiac research. Thus, it is now possible to conduct a rectal challenge with gluten protein in the doctor's office and get extremely reliable information that would allow the early and accurate diagnosis of celiac disease.

Highly sensitive and specific laboratory blood tests are more convenient and are already commercially available. They are being routinely used in Europe and the United States to screen for both gluten sensitivity and celiac disease. More than any other advancement in celiac disease, these tests are responsible for the increasing acceptance that gluten sensitivity is a very common illness, often responsible for an astounding variety of human diseases. In fact, there is talk in many research circles that, with some refinements, these screening tests may some day become the final diagnostic test of choice, entirely replacing intestinal biopsies.

REDEFINING GLUTEN SENSITIVITY

Unfortunately, elements of a century-old definition of celiac disease continue to limit diagnosis to those who show dramatic, advanced damage to the intestinal wall, representing only a small minority of those with celiac disease. The large majority of celiacs have silent or nonspecific, non-abdominal symptoms. Those who have specific antibodies against gluten circulating in their bloodstreams but do not show intestinal damage are frequently ignored, despite serious gluten-induced damage to a variety of other organs, tissues, and body systems.

For more than a decade now, world-renowned gastroenterologist, celiac-disease investigator, and author Dr. Michael N. Marsh, has been calling for renaming celiac disease "gluten sensitivity." World-renowned neurological researcher Dr. M. Hadjivassiliou, as a consequence of observing gluten sensitization in over half of his chronic neurological patients, has joined many other gastrointestinal researchers in calling for inclusion of non-celiac gluten sensitivity. Dr. Hadjivassiliou advocates that all patients with chronic neurological illnesses of unknown cause be routinely tested for gluten sensitivity. He recommends a gluten-free diet to all gluten-sensitive patients.

The broadened definition that many of these scientists are now advocating also includes routinely testing all patients for certain "genetic markers," such as human leukocyte antigen (HLA) markers; these are proteins found on the surface of our white blood cells that help identify susceptibility to dietary gluten.

A TREATMENT IN NEED OF CHANGE

The treatment of celiac disease has changed very little since the 1930s, with acceptance that wheat and related grains were at the root of celiac disease. While a strict gluten-free diet remains the only proven means of controlling this disease, recent research has shown that many celiac patients require a variety of additional tests and treatments to ensure optimum health.

The current unawareness of relevant research among U.S. and Canadian physicians dictates that comparatively few celiacs are ever diagnosed. Those few who are evaluated properly are usually underweight, complaining of abdominal symptoms, and have consulted a physician who is somewhat knowledgeable about celiac disease. These fortunate few are then referred to gastroenterologists more current in their knowledge about celiac disease. In turn, the gastroenterologist has the biopsies carefully examined by a pathologist who is trained to have a high level of suspicion for celiac disease. For the diagnosis of celiac disease to be made, all three physicians must be current in their research, recognize the importance of identifying celiac disease, and ever vigilant.

Given all the pitfalls, it is a bit more understandable why only one out of every forty of America's celiacs are diagnosed today. Yet it remains an unacceptable, deplorable situation. If not reversed soon, the continuing trend of underdiagnosis and delayed treatment may spell disaster for the American and Canadian health-care systems.

Blood tests for detecting gluten sensitivity and celiac disease and their dietary treatment impose little burden on our health-care systems. The cost of diagnosing and treating celiac disease, thereby preventing and reversing chronic pain syndromes, risk of cancers, osteoporosis, and complications of problem pregnancies, is comparatively cheap. This cost is significantly less than chemotherapy treatments, surgery to remove a tumor or fix a fractured hip, or long-term treatment of rheumatoid arthritis. More important, the cost in dollars pales next to all the unnecessary chronic, unremitting human suffering. Clearly, it is to the economic, social, and moral advantage of medical systems and health consumers everywhere to become aware of and much more vigilant in their search for celiac disease.

ADEQUATE FOLLOW-UP AND GUIDANCE BADLY NEEDED

Those diagnosed with celiac disease or gluten sensitivity are usually sent home with little helpful information. Newly diagnosed celiac patients are unlikely to be given information about the very high risk of celiac disease among their immediate family members, even though celiac disease is largely genetic and is transmitted from one generation to the next. First-degree family members are rarely encouraged to be tested and rarely notified of this potential danger to their health.

The extreme importance of strict, lifelong compliance with a gluten-free diet and the highly addictive nature of gluten are rarely adequately addressed. This explains in large part why the reported rate of strict gluten-free compliance is only about 50 percent.

Celiac patients are also not informed that they may have multiple delayed-onset food allergies. It is rare, indeed, that a celiac who continues to experience chronic symptoms after going gluten-free is tested for additional allergic foods. Yet, when celiac patients who remain symptomatic on a gluten-free diet are tested for additional food allergies, they often report good to excellent relief of symptoms with food allergen elimination.

Thirty-nine out of forty celiacs in the United States and Canada go undiagnosed. Most of them continue to struggle with ill health, uncertain about which way to turn, often blaming themselves for their compulsion to eat, chronic discomfort, lethargy, and fatigue. Many feel, after consulting with their doctors, that they have been summarily and abruptly dismissed with a symptom-chasing prescription drug or with reassurances implying in so many words that their problem is "all in their heads." Undetected celiacs die twice as frequently as non-celiacs, usually from cancers, but also osteoporotic hip fractures or complications of autoimmune diseases. Others endure avoidable, treatable chronic pain and disability. Learning to recognize gluten as a common underlying cause of many ills offers a sane, science-derived alternative explanation, giving hope to millions with chronic pain, that it is not their fault and that they can, at last, find permanent relief by dealing with the cause.

As you will learn in the following chapters, few of us really need tranquilizers, sleeping pills, antibiotics, hormone replacement, nonsteroidal anti-inflammatory drugs, or other pain-reducing medications to mask symptoms or our awareness of those symptoms. Instead, we need an effective, scientific, cause-oriented alternative to symptom-masking therapies. Many of you will find that alternative in a gluten-free diet.

When you finish reading this book, you will have a much better understanding of the dynamics that may be causing your disease, and indicators of potential, but preventable health problems that can result from consumption of grains.

The plague of the twentieth century was not cancer. Neither was it heart disease. Last century's plague was an insidious one that should have been recognized and treated long ago but wasn't. This plague remains poised, ready to harm many unwary victims. The signs of this growing, worldwide epidemic are apparent everywhere, to the initiated, including those who choose to read and carefully study this book. The worldwide epidemic is the plague of gluten gluttony, an overconsumption of wheat, rye, barley, and other gluten cereals by the vulnerable, genetically predisposed.

It is the explicit and recurring theme of this book that eating gluten grains drives much of mankind's chronic illness and that our escalating consumption of these grains is countering the many medical advances that are working to extend our lives. Through understanding the dynamics by which this occurs, our readers will be powerfully armed to protect themselves and their loved ones.

Grains and People:
An Evolutionary Mismatch

PLEASE NOTE: Although we draw much of our information for this chapter from the European–Middle East experience, this is perhaps even more valuable information for Asians, sub-Saharan Africans, Native Americans, Polynesians, and people of similar racial backgrounds because they have had significantly less time to adapt to consuming gluten. Europe and the Middle East are simply the birthplaces of wheat, rye, and barley cultivation, providing us with a rich source of information that has profound, worldwide relevance.

Our culture is steeped in pro-grain beliefs. You were probably taught that grains are a healthy food. They certainly played an important role in the development of Western civilization. Through religious beliefs, history classes in our schools, and our culinary traditions, grains have been given our cultural seal of approval in the absence of any scientific investigation. As a culture, we have simply ignored the growing body of evidence against grains, erroneously dismissing this information as applying only to a very few people or as a trivial concern voiced by hypochondriacs. Yet, there is a persuasive convergence of evidence against grains from several fields, including medicine, genetics, and archaeology.

In this chapter we offer a very brief exploration of that evidence, beginning with an archaeological overview of the evolution of preagricultural humans. Then we move to a discussion of the adoption of agriculture. We also provide information about how a leaky gut occurs among the genetically susceptible, often resulting from eating what is now our principal food—grains.

NATURAL SELECTION

Nature selects traits that allow individuals to survive long enough to reproduce. It may seem obvious, but if we die before we have children, our genes will not be passed on. For this reason, genetic diseases that fatally affect children are likely to decrease over generations. Further, youngsters are less likely to survive and pass on their genes if their parents do not survive long enough to help them through those first, most vulnerable years. Thus, the people whose parents live at least a few years beyond reproduction enjoy a selective advantage.

The impact of eating grains usually occurs well after reproduction, often in middle age. Therefore, the selection process puts only a little pressure on those who are gluten sensitive.

Our Four-Million-Year-Old Gene Pool

Our genetic heritage was shaped by the selection process. At least four million years ago, our branch of primates, called "upright" hominid, separated from great apes, gorillas, and chimpanzees. They have continued to evolve along their own branches of the primate tree, yet we continue to share more than 98 percent of our genetic heritage with the chimpanzee. This suggests just how slowly genetic change occurs in complex animals, such as humans, who must typically survive more than a decade before reproducing.

The diet of our closest genetic relative, the chimpanzee, supports the perspective that fruits and vegetables are healthful. It would be a mistake, however, to adopt a vegetarian perspective based on that rationale. Chimps do eat a great deal of fruit—when they are not eating each other! Recent observations suggest that cannibalism among chimpanzees is fairly common. Today's chimpanzee also hunts, kills, and eats small mammals. In fact, meat constitutes about 15 percent of the chimpanzee's diet. The notion that our evolutionary roots are strictly vegetarian is seriously flawed, even when viewed through the distorted lens of the contemporary chimpanzee's diet. The lesson, however, is an important one. Consumption of animal flesh has long played a significant role in the genetic past of our species.

Selective Advantage

In every species, the survival value of genetic mutations is constantly being tested by nature. Those new traits that continue from one generation to the next usually reflect an improved adaptation to the environment. Since the time we developed omnivorous teeth that functioned well for eating both vegetables and animals, our evolutionary heritage shifted to a greater general reliance on meat and internal organs. The human species and its forerunners survived, thrived, and evolved eating fish, meat, organs, vegetables, and fruit, for at least 1 million, and probably about 2.5 million years. Yet, humans have only been eating grains for the last twelve thousand years, showing the brevity of the span of evolutionary time during which we have been consuming grains. This means that humans have been eating meats and other animal parts 207 times longer than we have been eating grains. In other words, grain consumption has only taken place for less than one half of 1 percent of our evolutionary history.

Further, it is only those populations descended from the early farmers of the Middle East and southern Europe that have been eating significant quantities of cereal grains for as long as twelve thousand years. Most of the world's populations have had much less time to adapt to this very new food. Some groups of humans, including most aboriginal peoples throughout the world (such as Australian Aborigines and Native Americans) have had only a few centuries of exposure to gluten grains. In simplest terms, adaptation requires that only a minority of members of a particular species enjoys a selective advantage. The rest are culled from the gene pool. Adaptation is a ruthless process that can visit considerable suffering as it selects the most suitable genes for the current environment.

The 1993 Nobel Prize winner in chemistry, Kary Mullis, says that the "DNA molecules in our cells are our history." It is this genetic history that has shaped us. Our immune sensitivities and our nutritional requirements are decreed by the millions of years during which nature shaped our genes, our biochemistry, and our bodies. It did so through the interaction between the food in our environment and our ability to use it for energy, growth, and health. Thus, available foods shaped our genes, and our genes shaped our dietary requirements.

Modern humans were tall and robust when they spread through Africa, Europe, and Asia about forty thousand years ago. Like the Neanderthals and homo erectus before them, until the appearance of agriculture, the diet of modern humans was dominated by animal proteins and fats. There is considerable debate about the time at which we began to use cooking fires, with estimates ranging from two hundred thousand years ago to fifty thousand years ago.

By the time we started cooking our food, meat and internal organs already formed a major part of our diet. Our hunter-gatherer ancestors rarely, if ever, ate wild cereal grains prior to about 15,000 B.C. These grass seeds were very hard and could not provide any significant nutrition if eaten without grinding and cooking. Further, gluten grains, which are late arrivals to the human diet, lack many of the nutrients we need. They also contain substances that are harmful to us. These facts of grain composition clearly demonstrate both the short time we have been consuming them in any quantity and the poor suitability of grains as a dominant source of nutrients.

HUNTER-GATHERERS

We know that throughout most of recorded history humans usually lived short, difficult lives replete with famine, pestilence, and a high infant-mortality rate. We sometimes assume that this was also the case for their preagricultural, prehistoric hunter-gatherer ancestors, yet this is probably not the case. In fact, the available evidence from studies of modern hunter-gatherers suggests just the opposite.

Several isolated groups of hunter-gatherers were still in existence during the twentieth century. They had maintained their traditional lifestyle and were carefully observed by scientists like Vilhjalmur Stefansson. In addition to enjoying more leisure time than many people living in industrialized nations, such hunter-gatherers often lived long, healthy lives. There are many reasons to suspect that the same was true of our hunter-gatherer ancestors.

Prehistoric humans with crude tools may have been easy prey for the passing carnivore. It does seem likely that some of our distant ancestors provided large predators with the occasional meal, but the evidence also suggests that this was probably a two-way street. However, large, plant-eating animals like the mammoth, mastodon, bison, and elk were probably more important sources of our ancestors' food, if only because there was less confusion about who was hunting whom. Small animals, regardless of their feeding preferences, would also be attractive prey for early humans.

Archaeological evidence suggests that upright hominoids were using tools and hunting meat as much as 2.5 million years ago. Part of the evidence for these deductions comes from the tools used to butcher animals and extract their bone marrow. Authorities have attributed changes of tooth shape in these pre-humans to these dietary advances.

THE SWITCH TO AGRICULTURE—
AND ITS ADVANTAGES

Despite the health consequences of agriculture, it offered many advantages to early farmers. Grains can be stored for lengthy periods and with minimal technology. Although hunter-gatherer groups did store food, few foods are as amenable to long-term storage as grains. Further, it appears that humans were forced to seek alternative food sources due to the extinction or reduction of many of the world's large mammals. This dramatic decline among a host of large mammals occurred between ten thousand and twenty thousand years ago. Agriculture offered an alternative to the dwindling meat supply.

Early farmers would also appreciate the sense of physical comfort caused by these grains. Paradoxically, they provide this comfort through our inability to fully digest some parts of the grain. Undigested partial proteins, or peptides, found in gluten cereals have morphine-like properties, becoming potent drugs once they enter the bloodstream. Those who are at greatest risk from these foods often experience something akin to addiction due to the pleasant feelings caused by these exorphins, suggesting an origin for the phrase "comfort foods."

Another advantage of agriculture is that it allows people to develop settled communities, which usually resulted in specialization of labor. More substantial homes and fortresses were built, providing better protection from the elements, predators, and aggressive neighbors. Farming also supports more people on a given area land, which confers yet another defensive advantage. There is little doubt that agriculture offered many attractions to the earliest farmers.

Adopting agriculture may have provided humans with a storable food surplus, yet it had many negative genetic health impacts. Many explanations have been offered for this change in health and stature associated with grain consumption. Some suspect that it was famine and/or disease that first prompted humans to begin cultivating and eating cereal grains, blaming these other factors for the decline in health associated with farming. These arguments pale in light of recent medical and scientific discoveries.

Our agricultural ancestors became smaller, their bones became weaker and more diseased, and the size of their brains diminished. Human brain size, based on head circumference, has diminished approximately 11 percent since the advent of agricultural societies. Modern European hunter-gatherer men and women stood five to six inches taller than farmers of a few generations later. Only recently, as a result of DNA analysis, has it become evident that the shorter farmers were actually descendants of the taller hunter-gatherers. There are many archaeological excavations throughout the world that indicate this cereal-associated dynamic, regardless of when agriculture was begun. Clearly, the nutrient-rich hunter-gatherer lifestyle is most likely the factor that decreed the five to six inches difference in stature.

If we take celiac disease as a model for other forms of gluten sensitivity, the evidence clearly suggests that eating gluten in increasingly larger amounts was, in all likelihood, the primary cause of these reductions in bone health, stature, and brain size experienced by the first farmers. Diminution of brain size and brain weight has been reported to be overrepresented in untreated older celiacs. Virtually every adult-diagnosed patient with celiac disease demonstrates significant reductions in bone density compared with age-equivalent averages. Short stature is another common feature of untreated celiac disease. Given today's medical evidence, there can now be little doubt that such changes among early farmers were the direct result of eating grains. The evolutionary pressures began with the first gluten-containing meal. We started trimming a few members of the gene pool with each succeeding generation of farmers.

GRAINS EVOLVED TOO

The negative impact of grains on early farmers was comparatively reduced to that of today. Gluten content is much greater in today's grains. That may be best understood through the forces of evolution that shaped these grains. Many of the detrimental changes to grains are the result of human choices or actions, rather than natural selection. This process, although probably unintentional at first, was partly the result of planting and harvesting practices.

When ripe, the wild cereal seeds would fall off the stalk and seed the next year's grass. Fully ripened seeds are only briefly available on the stalk before falling to the ground. The selective gathering of these mature seeds would be inefficiently time consuming for hungry hunter-gatherers. But due to the development of modern farming techniques, today's crops ripen fairly uniformly because of the many centuries of selection that accompany seasonal harvesting.

Rapid genetic change may be induced, whether among humans or other species, if it bears on reproduction. Such change can be quite rapid in a plant that reproduces annually and that is specifically selected for reproduction. In other words, undesirable genetic traits in cereal grains, such as the grains falling off the stalk prematurely or ripening later than the others, would be quickly eliminated.

Further spread of agriculture required additional evolutionary change for successful grain cultivation in harsher climates. The east-west spread of cereal farming from the Middle East's Fertile Crescent to Southern Europe occurred quite quickly and required little or no genetic change to grains. This is due to similarities of day length, climate, predators, and diseases at similar latitudes. On the other hand, cultivation in more northerly latitudes of Europe required some important changes in genetic traits.

Wheat grown further north must ripen during a shorter number of longer days and must be able to withstand early frost. Northern grains were also faced with new predators and diseases. Adaptation to more northerly latitudes is at the root of an important development of this wheat seed. Gluten is a group of storage proteins. In order for seeds to germinate, they need nutrients that are contained within the seed. Northern grains must contain relatively more gluten and other storage proteins as they must make the most of the shorter growing season and germinate in the more hostile environment.

Wheat, rye, and barley grains, all members of the grass family, contain particular types of nutrients, or storage proteins, which are very difficult for humans to digest but are ideal for the germinating grain. One group of these storage proteins is commonly called gliadin, and it is thought to do most of the damage to human intestines in cases of gluten sensitivity and celiac disease. Glutenins are another group of storage proteins found in gluten. Glutenins are thought to be associated with autoimmune skin diseases and perhaps certain cases of asthma. Digestion of these storage proteins requires very specific digestive enzymes, which most of us lack. The combined increase in storage proteins and the absence of the enzymes required to digest them have created a problem that is further escalated by the appeal of these resilient northerly grains.

This increased gluten content associated with northerly cultivation is highly prized for its baking characteristics. Heat resistance, elasticity, and malleability due to high gluten content make baked products that are more attractive to the eye, with a lighter texture. The Canadian Wheat Marketing Board proudly guarantees and annually delivers millions of tons of Canadian Hard wheat to major food manufacturers, frequently winning international awards and acclaim for its "superior" quality wheat with increased gluten content. The very properties that make this grain more attractive for culinary uses also increase its threat to human health. It is an unfortunate trend with a very old heritage.

THE SPREAD OF ROMAN GRAIN

Our earliest exposure to grains was in southeastern Europe, where the gluten content of grain was comparatively small. Agriculture spread fairly quickly to the west, but movement to the north was slower. Although agriculture was fairly widespread by the time of the rise of the Roman Empire, the Romans aided the development of efficient grain cultivation throughout most of Europe. However, the Romans did not conquer every area. Parts of Ireland, Scotland, and Finland managed to evade Roman rule. Many of the people in these areas have been consuming only small quantities of grains until very recently. For example, in Denmark during the 1950s, many Danes considered wheat bread to be a special treat due to the fact that wheat does not grow well in Denmark. North American natives have had a similarly brief exposure to gluten. Genetic differences between these groups and those who have had a longer period to adapt to gluten may identify some of the most threatening elements of grain consumption.

GENETICS, THE UNIFYING THREAD

The field of genetics has bridged the gaps between various biological sciences. Similarly, a growing understanding of the interactions between evolution and food sensitivities offers to unify the study of the diseases of civilization. Thanks to DNA analysis, we can look back into the distant past and see where we have come from. This also allows us to better understand some of the dietary practices from our prehistory; the practices that have shaped our needs and capacities today.

Because gluten sensitivity is often a silent disease in its early stages, most people who suffer from it have few identifiable symptoms or illnesses until adulthood. Yet, over a lifetime, those with celiac disease are about twice as likely to die prematurely. This increase in deaths is usually from common complications of celiac disease such as intestinal cancers, osteoporotic hip fractures, insulin-dependent diabetes, etc. A trait such as this that reduces the likelihood of survival should be found in fewer people of each succeeding generation. However, such early deaths usually occur after reproductive years, therefore passing on the genes that determine gluten sensitivity. It is thus that this trait continues to be passed from one generation to the next despite the development and increased reliance on cereal cultivation. Because of the survival disadvantages it imposes, mostly in the areas of infertility and recurring miscarriage, gluten sensitivity should slowly diminish in numbers over many generations of exposure to gluten-containing grains, especially when gluten content is continually on the rise. However, many of us may be unwilling to pay the price exacted by the slow pace of natural selection. Reverting to a diet free of gluten may be a preferable choice if you are one of those who are genetically susceptible.

WHAT'S IN YOUR GENES?

The part of the immune system that is unique to each person is made up of human leukocyte antigens (HLA). HLA are associated with the progression of infectious diseases and the susceptibility to an incredibly wide range of chronic, noninfectious diseases, including celiac disease. In commercially available genetic blood tests, these HLA features are identified in celiac patients by the proteins found on the surface of certain white blood cells. For example, on the outer surface of some of these white blood cells, HLA proteins named DQ2 and DQ8 are found in more than 90 and 94 percent of those with celiac disease, respectively. HLA-B8 is also common in celiac disease and is found in about 80 percent of celiac patients.

The appearance of these HLA proteins in the people of a particular population is a good indicator of the time that a region has been growing gluten grains. In Europe, HLA-B8 is found in less than 10 percent of the people living in the area where wheat was first cultivated thousands of years ago. Yet, it is found in more than 30 percent of the populations living in the far northwest of Europe, including the west of Ireland, Iceland, and parts of Scandinavia, especially Finland, where wheat cultivation was introduced much later and where historically such crops did not fare as well.

The genetic trait that confers gluten sensitivity has remained in the human gene pool for a very long time, causing untold, unnecessary suffering as it continues undetected. In the minority of cases where gluten does interfere with reproduction, the impact can be heartbreaking and extremely stressful. For instance, there is a high prevalence of infertility, regardless of which spouse has celiac disease. If the expectant mother is an untreated celiac, she is more likely to experience recurring miscarriages, premature births, and low birth weights. Italian obstetricians have recently found undetected celiac disease to be so common among women who have problem pregnancies that they are advocating that all pregnant women entering their clinics be routinely screened with blood tests.

With today's scientific and archaeological advances, we now know many of the diseases that accompany the shift to high cereal consumption. Those populations exposed to gluten within the last few centuries are demonstrating the devastating impact of adoption of these grains into the human diet. One need only look at the epidemic of diabetes, thyroid disease, cancer, iron deficiency, malnutrition, and major depression among many aboriginal groups just recently introduced to a gluten-rich diet to deduce the horrible impact on genetically naïve populations consuming these cereals. If we are to deal effectively with this health threat, we need to understand how proteins are digested and the difference this can make.

Making Essential Nutrients Out of Proteins

The building blocks for proteins such as gluten are amino acids. Food proteins are made up of twenty common amino acids, eight of which are absolutely essential. They must be found in what we eat because we are unable to manufacture them from other nutrients. Several more amino acids are "conditionally essential." Glutamine and arginine, for instance, are conditionally essential amino acids. During chronic disease or stress, we need more conditionally essential amino acids than our bodies are able to manufacture.

All of these different amino acids are bound together in specific sequences, making up protein chains, or polypeptides, frequently composed of hundreds, sometimes thousands, of separate amino acid molecules.

Digestion of Dietary Protein

Optimal digestion involves disintegration of these large, complex dietary proteins into smaller particles. Sometimes proteins are reduced into their smallest units of single, free amino acids. Even peptides composed of two or three amino acids need not be digested further. These small molecules can easily be transported through the cells of the intestinal

wall, where they are absorbed into the bloodstream as nutrients. Optimally, about 70 percent of digested proteins are absorbed as small peptides, while the remaining 30 percent are absorbed as free amino acids.
Usually, the healthy digestive system wastes the undigested and partly digested proteins as fecal matter.

Some bonds between the amino acids that form gluten proteins are
extremely resistant to intestinal digestion. While some individuals produce a liver enzyme capable of digesting gluten, many do not. It is not yet
clear if the presence of these enzymes provides protection from gluten
sensitivity, but it does seem probable. For the many who lack these digestive enzymes, grains need much more processing than the foods that are
common to a hunter-gatherer's diet. Even after grinding, cooking, and the
many assaults of processing and digestion, some of these gluten proteins
remain stubbornly intact. The mucus that lines our intestines usually pro-
tects our bloodstream from these stubborn proteins.

Undigested Grain Proteins Spell Trouble

Ideally, we would waste all of these often-indigestible proteins and go
on to our next meal unharmed. However, there is a lot of evidence to
show that somewhere between 15 and 42 percent of the general population are absorbing some of these undigested and partly digested gluten
proteins into their blood by passing them between the cells that line
the intestinal wall. Once in the bloodstream, antibody production often
follows, causing inflammation at the site where these proteins are being
leaked. The chemicals released as a result of inflammation cause even
greater permeability, and a self-perpetuating cycle is established.

This abnormal intestinal permeability, aptly labeled "the leaky gut
syndrome," results from a variety of causes, including gluten sensitivity.
Because gluten proteins have been shown to damage many internal organs and tissues on contact, absorption of these partly digested proteins
is a major threat to one's health even in the absence of specific antibodies against gliadins or other gluten proteins.

Our Tennis-Court-Sized Intestinal Lining

As proteins move along the digestive tract, they come in contact with the mucosal lining of the small intestine, which serves at least three important functions:

1. It releases many gut hormones and enzymes that stimulate or aid digestion and intestinal immune function. These hormones also communicate with the brain and heart;
2. It absorbs health-promoting nutrients from food;
3. It acts as a selective barrier, blocking absorption of undigested or partly digested proteins, as well as toxins, anti-nutrients, bacteria, yeast, and parasites.

The importance and extent of these three functions is reflected in the size of the mucosa of a healthy small intestine. If it was spread out and flattened to show its entire absorptive surface, it would be larger than the playing surface of a tennis court!

Like the skin, our intestinal lining serves as a protective barrier against the environment. It has the highest concentration and mass of immune cells in the entire human body. Unlike the skin, however, the lining is only one cell thick. These tens of billions of highly specialized cells are replaced very rapidly, normally about every seventy-two hours. Imagine growing an entirely new skin every three days—which is just what healthy intestines do. Curiously, this extraordinarily dynamic selective barrier is the first to be cannibalized and destroyed when we're exposed to any form of severe stress such as major surgery, radiation, chemotherapy, ultra-endurance sports, severe burns, and, in some cases, gluten. Recent research conducted by Loren Cordain, a researcher at Colorado State University, has also reported several anti-nutrients, psychoactive substances, and other non-gluten agents discovered in cereals that can damage the human intestinal wall.

YOU MAY BE ASKING: WHAT DOES ALL THAT MEAN TO ME?

If you are a member of that large segment of the U.S. population that is at greater risk of having a leaky gut, or if you undergo one of the many events that can cause temporary leakage, you are inviting undigested gluten into your bloodstream. This assumes, of course, that you are eating what has become a normal diet that includes wheat, rye, and/or barley. Since our digestive tract is designed to absorb nutrients through the cells in the intestinal lining, not through gaps between these cells, when absorption occurs between the cells, the protective function of the intestinal tract is thwarted.

Under such circumstances, you not only risk absorbing undigested and partly digested proteins from gluten, food additives, other dietary proteins, and toxins into your blood, you also increase your risk of infectious disease. Bacteria that is normally held within the intestine and not associated with infection may be absorbed whole into the blood, depositing in distant tissue, causing infections and autoimmune reactions. This process is called "bacterial translocation." Other bacteria, perhaps from the food supply, may also be allowed access to your bloodstream. Clearly, a wide range of ailments can develop as the result of a leaky gut.

OUR IMMUNE SYSTEMS

Occasional or chronic leakage of proteins into the blood can take varying periods of time to produce a wide range of signs and symptoms. It is thus difficult to identify the cause of many resulting illnesses. Even making the connection between symptoms and a particular food can be difficult. Delayed reactions to foods, from several hours to several days, are common and are called "delayed-type hypersensitivity." The delay is caused by the time needed for these foods to be processed in the stomach, released into the intestine, absorbed into the circulatory system, and an immune response to be activated. Some elements of the immune system require as much as seventy-two hours to begin acting against such invaders.

Gluten, if allowed to remain in circulation, while also constantly being replenished by the diet, will cause damage to a variety of tissues and body organs. Gluten sensitivity has long been seen as an immune system error. However, gluten will also injure many human tissues. Since it will cause this tissue damage, whether it gained entry into the blood through gluten sensitivity or by some other means, an immune reaction to these proteins may not reflect a flawed immune system. The critical issue appears to be whether gluten gains entry into the blood. Therefore, celiac disease represents only a small sector of the range of human immune reactions to the presence of gluten either in the intestinal tract or in the bloodstream because about 15 percent of the population demonstrates some type of immune reaction to gluten proteins.

The first time the immune system is exposed to a particular foreign protein, there is a delay before an immune response is fully mounted. Following that first exposure, our immune system will often work rapidly to seek out and destroy this invader whenever it appears again. This is the result of memory cells that were developed against that foreign protein during the first exposure. This occurs whether these proteins are in the form of a bacterial, fungal, parasitical, or viral infection, or in the form of an allergen.

Thus, among the genetically susceptible, after the first leakage of gluten into the blood, every time gluten is present in the intestine, a healthy immune system identifies the presence of gluten through intestinal sensors, and cascades of immune responses follow. Many researchers exploring gluten sensitivity have expressed the notion that the vigorous immune response mounted by people with celiac disease probably enjoyed a selective advantage in preagricultural societies. This may be the result of a form of vaccination.

EARLY VACCINATION

Most vaccinations inject dead infectious agents into the bloodstream. This will sensitize the immune system. The "invader" proteins, although dead, result in the creation of memory cells, so that the next time these proteins are detected in the blood, a rapid reaction can be mounted. Such subsequent reactions are usually so rapid that we often do not develop any symptoms and are probably unaware of the return of this invader.

A genetic inclination to develop a leaky gut may have served a similar function among hunter-gatherers. Infants fed small amounts of other foods, in addition to suckling the mother's milk, would be swallowing many bacteria. Some of the bacteria from these foods, and some from the breast and/or hands that fed them, would pass through the stomach and into the intestine. Although likely to be killed by the acid environment of the stomach and maternal antibodies in the milk, some proteins would predictably remain intact to be absorbed through the intestinal wall and into the bloodstream. Here, a very early, effective form of vaccination might develop.

OUR CHANGING FOOD SUPPLY

Our food supply is narrowing. It is a trend that we have continued since adopting agriculture, moving away from animal fats and proteins toward a cereal-dominated diet. Today, few of us consume meat from a wide variety of wild animals. Our diet is restricted to a small variety of domestic meats. Neither do we liberally choose from over three hundred species of edible plants. Today, we are restricted to a very small selection of twenty to thirty vegetables and fruits, and most of us choose from a much narrower range dictated solely by preference. The majority of our calories and much of our dietary protein come from cereal grains, mostly wheat, rice, corn (maize), and cow's milk products—foods never touched by most humans as recently as just a few thousand years ago. Our genetics are unchanged, but our diet has been radically transformed, and therein lies the rub.

Dairy and gluten-grain products combine to make up the top six foods we now eat. Yet cow's milk and wheat are two of the most commonly reported allergens in the world. With individuals genetically predisposed to food allergies and gluten sensitivity, eating these same nonancestral, genetically incompatible foods in large quantities day in and day out, is it any wonder that so many people suffer from chronic food sensitivities?

Types of Celiac Disease
and Non-Celiac Gluten Sensitivity

Y ou may be wondering why it is important to devote an entire chapter to the various types of celiac disease and gluten sensitivity. In chapter 1, we discussed a number of ways that gluten can affect the body. Yet, most research attention involving gluten has been focused on only one expression of gluten sensitivity—celiac disease. Because of the amount of information that exists about celiac disease, it does provide the best window through which to examine the broader realm of gluten sensitivity. Still, it is important to emphasize that the people with celiac disease represent only a small portion of the population that is adversely affected by gluten. Applying assumptions and generalizations about one form of gluten sensitivity to all gluten-related conditions is potentially dangerous. In this chapter we offer information that will help you avoid this pitfall and identify the differing types of gluten sensitivity.

In order to better understand the various types of gluten sensitivity, we will discuss classic celiac disease, atypical celiac disease, silent or asymptomatic celiac disease, latent celiac disease, non-celiac gluten sensitivity, and examples of specific ailments affected by gluten. While these conditions all respond positively to a gluten-free diet, there is great variability in how they should be managed in addition to compliance with the diet. Each form of gluten sensitivity has its own unique characteristics, symptoms, risks, and degrees of response to treatment. Understanding the range of conditions will reduce the risk of leaping to risky assumptions about your health. This chapter will also aid in deciding whether or not a strict gluten-free diet is worth a try.

There are also some specific non-celiac ailments, conditions, and treatments that can be helped by a gluten-free diet, although the reasons for its benefit are not yet well understood. These conditions include intestinal injuries caused by chemical and radiation therapies, AIDS, and food allergies. It is important not to confuse these conditions with celiac disease, despite the shared feature of clinical improvement on a gluten-free diet.

There is still considerable variability and uncertainty related to non-celiac gluten sensitivity. If only for this reason, it is important that individuals at risk should have enough information to make an informed decision for themselves. The risks associated with various forms of gluten sensitivity are not identical to those of untreated celiac disease. However, we are forced to base many of our deductions on experience and celiac-specific research, beginning with the most commonly recognized form.

CLASSIC CELIAC DISEASE

Classic celiac disease is a condition that will be familiar to most physicians and other health-care practitioners. A very limited view of celiac disease develops where understanding is limited to classic celiac presentation. Yet this form has been extremely popular in teaching centers for the last forty years or so. Unfortunately, even with its near universal acceptance, when a patient demonstrates the signs and symptoms of classic celiac disease, an accurate diagnosis still takes an average of eleven years in the United States and Canada. It also frequently requires visiting a number of doctors before it is even suspected. This is in large part due to the outdated notion that celiac disease is quite rare. Celiac disease is sometimes not sought due to the faulty belief that it is a fairly harmless condition that can reasonably wait while other more harmful diseases are ruled out.

The patient with classic celiac disease typically arrives at the doctor's office appearing pale and lethargic; complaining of diarrhea, excessive gas, and abdominal pain; and showing signs of malnutrition, a low-grade

I am a midlife "baby boomer" currently living in New England. As a very early teen, after I had fainted a couple of times, my family doctor told my parents that I had iron deficiency anemia. Since I was a teenage girl and just starting to menstruate, the doctor attributed my anemia to excessive blood loss during my menstrual cycles. Over the next thirty-five years, at least four different doctors diagnosed me with severe iron deficiency anemia of unknown cause. I managed to increase my iron by taking supplements and eating high-iron foods, but as soon as I went off supplemental iron, my anemia recurred.

In the mid-1980s I began to lose weight, going from 125 to under 110 pounds (at a height of five feet, six inches), and I felt increasingly fatigued. My fatigue and inability to concentrate contributed to my having withdrawn from two doctoral programs. Since the early 1990s, I complained of increasingly severe lower back pain, leading to a referral to an endocrinologist. I had developed premature osteoporosis. In the summer of 1997, hip pain and mobility problems resulted in the diagnosis of a very rare bone fracture in my right hip. In the summer of 1997, I began experiencing intermittent GI bleeding.

By February 1998, with continued GI bleeding, bloating, abdominal pain, and loss of appetite, my primary care physician referred me to a gastroenterologist. By that time, I weighed 90 pounds, and, although I didn't know it, I had lost over two inches in height due to osteoporosis. Within ten minutes, after hearing

> my current complaints and medical history, the gastroenterologist told me that she was quite certain I had celiac sprue. Her diagnosis was confirmed by both blood tests and a biopsy. I went on a gluten-free diet. Within three months, blood tests showed that my iron levels were within normal limits, and, staying on a strict gluten-free diet, I have not experienced anemia in nearly three years. My weight has also reached a more normal range; I have been able to gain more than 15 pounds and keep it between 108 and 114 most of the time, except when I'm under stress.
>
> *Pat S.*

fever, and a bloated stomach. A few pointed questions will soon reveal that the patient's stools often float and have a particularly unpleasant odor, suggesting a high-fat content. Although one might expect that such dramatic signs and symptoms would lead to a rapid diagnosis, this is usually not the case. These classic recognizable manifestations of celiac disease are the exception, not the rule, of celiac patients. Those with atypical symptoms are very unlikely to get an accurate diagnosis.

ATYPICAL CELIAC DISEASE

Many cases of celiac disease present with a single symptom or with symptoms that are unlikely to be connected with celiac disease. Examples of such atypical presentations range from life-threatening cavities in the lung wall to severe cases of rheumatoid arthritis to headaches that just won't go away. It is a rare practitioner who suspects celiac disease when faced with such conditions. Yet, there are many dozens of examples of such atypical symptoms. In fact, we have identified well over 150 medical conditions and symptoms, most of which should be categorized as atypical celiac disease. A listing is provided in appendix D.

The further one looks into medical literature, the more difficult it becomes to ignore the possibility of celiac disease in association with almost any condition or symptom. Celiac disease simply cannot be ruled out without testing, and those who do not suspect, do not test. Even those who have a high level of suspicion of celiac disease will be misled if they rely on classical symptoms to suggest celiac disease.

SILENT OR ASYMPTOMATIC CELIAC DISEASE

Any search for celiac disease based on the presence of symptoms will miss most cases. This is because nearly half are clinically silent. Over half of all biopsy-proven celiacs have no abdominal symptoms at the time of diagnosis, even though intestinal damage has been occurring for years.

One might argue that if the patient has no symptoms, the patient should be left alone until aggravating symptoms develop. Tragically, as discussed in hundreds of medical journals, the first, most common presenting symptom of silent celiac disease may be cancer. There is a similarly grave risk of developing other chronic, potentially life-shortening ailments that so often follow undetected, untreated celiac disease. For this majority of celiac victims, blood testing is their best, perhaps their only hope for diagnosis. But this risk can be reversible if a gluten-free diet is begun early enough. The risk of malignancy may actually be greater among silent celiacs because so few of them are likely to be diagnosed and hence have not had the opportunity to reduce their astronomically high cancer risk through a gluten-free diet.

LATENT CELIAC DISEASE

There are many cases in which celiac disease is suspected but no intestinal damage can be found; yet, months or years later, frank celiac disease is found. One commonly sees this with first-degree family members of celiacs and in recently diagnosed insulin-dependent diabetics. The initial biopsy is negative, only to turn positive six months to three years later. This latency and dormancy demonstrate a phenomenon that has long been recognized as a disturbing feature of this disease. Not only do the symptoms of celiac disease wax and wane but also the damage to the intestinal wall seems to vary.

This has several important implications. It suggests that we should treat any person with positive blood tests, but negative biopsies, as potential celiacs. More specifically, it questions whether or not these "false positive" anti-gliadin blood tests are meaningful or helpful. It also reveals a problem with intestinal biopsies as a diagnostic tool. As long as we accept the notion that such biopsies provide a gold standard for diagnosis, it should alert us to the need for regular and repeated testing.

NON-CELIAC GLUTEN SENSITIVITY

A similarly broad range can be found in non-celiac gluten sensitivity. Simply put, those people who have a nonspecific injury to the intestinal mucosa that leaks food proteins and toxins into the blood but do not have the damaged villi and/or increased intestinal immune cells found in untreated celiac disease can be said to have non-celiac gluten sensitivity. Identification of this form of gluten sensitivity is as simple as getting a blood test for specific antibodies. Non-celiac gluten sensitivity afflicts about 20 percent of the American and Canadian population and, along with the telling elevated antibodies against gluten, can be found in most of the same ailments that are overrepresented among untreated celiacs.

DERMATITIS HERPETIFORMIS—AN EXAMPLE OF BOTH CELIAC AND NON-CELIAC GLUTEN SENSITIVITY

Dermatitis herpetiformis is a lifelong gluten-sensitive skin disease. Also known as Duhring's disease, this fascinating subgroup of celiac disease

Thirty-Three Years of Itching
Ends with a Gluten-Free Diet

I developed an itchy rash starting on my elbows my senior year in college. Over several months the rash spread to my knees and different parts of the rest of my body. This was in the mid-1960s. I visited many doctors, an allergist, and several dermatologists over the years.

Over thirty-three years after the rash started, I happened to see an article in *Prevention* magazine describing the case of a woman with dermatitis herpetiformis. I had never heard of celiac disease, dermatitis herpetiformis, or gluten before. I got on the Internet, and within fifteen minutes I knew that I had this gluten-induced skin disease. It was a classic case. I immediately went on a gluten-free diet, and on the third day, I stopped itching for the first time in over thirty years.

I then saw a gastroenterologist. I looked too healthy to be a celiac. He agreed to do a blood test, and after a little research he agreed to do a biopsy. Both the biopsy and blood test were positive for celiac disease. It took a few months for the rash to totally clear up. I also had a number of digestive and gynecological problems go away.

Barb W.

shows itself primarily on the skin. The most common locations for these lesions are the back of the knees, buttocks, elbows, and the face.

Sometimes in the form of a rash and sometimes in the form of multiple pimplelike lesions, dermatitis herpetiformis is usually extremely itchy. The rash or lesion is usually symmetrical—that is, if there are one or two itchy lesions on one buttock or leg, there will soon be the same number in the same approximate location on the other side of the face. Dermatitis herpetiformis lesions often develop following exposure to sunlight or iodine. A primitive and unreliable means of diagnosing this condition is to soak a patch of fabric in iodine and tape it to the skin. If a lesion developed, dermatitis herpetiformis was diagnosed. Today's diagnostic procedures are much more accurate.

About 75 percent of individuals with this gluten-induced skin condition show intestinal damage on biopsy. It is important to recognize that the increased risks of cancer and other sequelae of dermatitis herpetiformis are about the same as those associated with untreated celiac disease. Many researchers consider dermatitis herpetiformis to be a skin manifestation of celiac disease and maintain that improved testing techniques will reveal gluten-induced intestinal damage in all cases of this skin disease.

There is little to be gained, other than convenience, by continuing to eat gluten in the context of dermatitis herpetiformis. Yet, few dermatologists recognize this disease, and all too often those who do continue to recommend drug treatment in place of dietary intervention, oblivious to the danger of cancer, which is only preventable with a gluten-free diet. Such drug treatment may control the symptoms of this disease; however, the insidious, gluten-induced damage to tissues, organs, and body systems will continue.

RANGES OF SENSITIVITY IN CELIAC DISEASE

An important consideration, especially when developing an understanding of celiac disease, is to recognize that, while the health risks appear to remain constant for people with celiac disease, the symptoms do not. This means that some people with celiac disease will be exquisitely sensitive to the slightest quantity of gluten, while others may eat significant quantities of gluten with little or no apparent response.

On the surface, this might suggest that some celiacs can eat gluten safely. But the research does not support that perspective. This is an area where we still have a great deal to learn, but it appears that there is variability in how much of the intestine is affected by gluten. According to one report, less than one gram of gluten daily is sufficient to perpetuate intestinal damage in a celiac. The range and variability of symptoms also suggest that there are many individual differences from one patient to the next, particularly regarding the region of the small intestine that is affected by gluten.

An Extreme Reaction to Gluten

In 1991 I started having digestive symptoms and losing weight. My doctor started testing. Eventually, during a visit to the doctor, I mentioned that I seemed to feel better in the morning if I ate Cream of Rice cereal. The doctor mentioned that there was a rare disorder called celiac sprue and urged me to try a gluten-free diet. I did start feeling better for a while—but not for long. The weight loss continued. I started becoming "clumsy." I'd drop things and seemed to trip over my own feet. My hands and feet began to feel like they were rubber rather than skin. I lost more weight. With more meds and continued testing, I had so much abdominal pain that it was difficult to function. I was exhausted all the time, and I started having panic attacks. I lost 85 of 215 pounds. I am a tall woman—but I looked like a concentration camp survivor. I also experienced spontaneous bruising. I could watch as a spot on my arm or leg would swell, hurt like heck, and then turn vibrant purple.

In January 1992 I was hospitalized. I could barely use my left hand. I was cold all the time. It was all I could do to stay awake. I was having severe head pains and still losing weight after more testing. A psychiatrist was called in. He announced I had what was then called a major affective disorder (depression). I was counseled for anorexia. My guts hurt, my bowel movements were foul, and I was tired of trying to stay alive.

Though still on a gluten-free diet, I was worse than when the doctor first suggested celiac disease. My salvation came when a hospital dietitian was monitoring my food intake due to suspicions of anorexia. The dietitian brought me a photocopy of a booklet about celiac disease. On the last page there was a blurb about making sure your medications had been checked to assure they did not contain gluten. A call to the pharmacist confirmed that nine of the eleven medications I was taking contained gluten. As soon as I stopped taking all but my thyroid medications, I started getting better.

Slowly I got my energy back. I started feeling human again. My body had deteriorated so much that it had been devouring itself in an attempt to find protein. I was starving to death, and if this had continued much longer, my body would have not been able to restore itself. I was lucky.

Deni W.

APPLICATION OF CELIAC RESEARCH TO GLUTEN SENSITIVITY

Only a little research has been conducted in the broader realm of gluten sensitivity. We therefore rely heavily on the research into celiac disease to deduce risks and prognoses. Researchers working in this area commonly test for, and report, levels of anti-gliadin antibodies among their subjects. We have therefore generalized findings from celiac disease to the larger population of gluten-sensitive people. There are several problems with our approach. It is impossible to say that all individuals who are gluten sensitive will suffer the same risk of a given disease as those with celiac disease. This possibility of a reduced risk raises some important questions. Just how strictly should we exclude gluten from the diet? What are the economic and social implications of gluten exclusion? Despite these questions, some of the best-informed scientists investigating celiac disease have arrived at a position similar to the one we are taking. They argue for a shift away from the current focus on celiac disease, to explore gluten sensitivity more fully.

The world-renowned researcher Michael N. Marsh has argued for redefining celiac disease and changing the name to "gluten sensitivity." He has also pressed for defining this disease exclusively on the basis of immune reactions to gluten. Dr. Marsh limits his discussion of the immune responses to gluten that can be identified from changes in the intestinal wall following direct contact with gluten.

On the other hand, others have clearly shown that many types of human tissues are damaged when they come in contact with gluten. If we are mounting an immune response to gluten, it is reasonable to conclude that we are leaking some of these proteins or derivative peptides into our blood. If they are reaching the bloodstream, then a wide range of tissue damage is predictable.

Rather than ignoring chronically ill, non-celiac gluten-sensitive individuals who show no tissue damage on biopsy, we suspect that any and all identifiable immune responses to gluten should be recognized as dangerous. The evidence strongly suggests that everyone mounting such an immune response should be encouraged to strictly exclude all gluten from his or her diet.

Proactively Determining
Your Risk

Gluten grains are a leading cause of many ailments. Avoiding gluten prevents and often reverses these diseases. Should you passively wait for the signs and symptoms of disease to arrive before taking action? There are many cases of apparently healthy individuals who seem to suddenly succumb to celiac-associated cancers, autoimmune diseases, or other serious celiac-associated ailments, although there is little prior indication of the underlying disease.

Fortunately, there are rational alternatives. With the help of simple, affordable blood tests that are available to all health consumers, you can now determine your genetic makeup and the presence or absence of antibodies indicating gluten sensitization and celiac disease. In addition, armed with the information in this book, you can examine your own family and medical history for evidence of a gluten problem.

None of these sources can conclusively diagnose celiac disease or gluten sensitivity. However, the patterns formed by an orderly examination of information drawn from all of these areas will reveal your own unique risk of developing one or more gluten-induced ailments.

Information on relevant testing and when to eliminate gluten from one's diet will follow in later chapters. Understanding what signs indicate risk and how to evaluate your own unique pattern of risk is the most important first step toward preventing, arresting, and/or reversing gluten-induced illness. The cause of many symptoms and complaints often becomes obvious in hindsight, yet it remains obscure to those of us who still consider wheat to be the staff of life.

SELF-EXAMINATION

In your search for clues and warning signs, the first place to look is within. You know your own moods better than anyone. You know your cravings or addictions. You know your own habits. You are probably more aware of your appearance and stature, too. Who could know your sleep requirements and energy levels better than you? And what about your perceptions, minor pains, abdominal bloating, and your susceptibility to colds or the flu? Each of us is our own best expert when it comes to ourselves.

Questions to Ask Yourself Now, Rather than Later

1. Is there anyone in your immediate family who is a proven celiac or is gluten sensitive?

   ❑ yes ❑ no

   If yes, you are at high risk of having or developing gluten problems.

2. Are you or is any member of your immediate family a victim of an autoimmune disease such as insulin-dependent diabetes, autoimmune thyroid disease, or Addison's (adrenal) disease?

   ❑ yes ❑ no

All of these conditions are commonly found in celiacs and their family members.

3. What are your eating habits? Do you have food cravings?

   ❑ yes   ❑ no

   If so, what foods do you crave?_____
   If dairy products or foods with high levels of gluten are on your list, we suggest that you seek testing for celiac disease and food allergies. Because some of the partial proteins from gluten and dairy products can be highly addictive, if they are regularly absorbed into the circulation, cravings for these foods are cause for concern.

4. After meals, do you often feel bloated and uncomfortable? Do you have to loosen your belt? Is breathing more difficult? Is the bloating often associated with an inexplicable gain of two to five pounds within a twenty-four-hour period?

   ❑ yes   ❑ no

5. Have you ever had one or more bouts of severe abdominal cramping?

   ❑ yes   ❑ no

   If you have celiac disease or gluten sensitivity, such cramping can sometimes be so severe that it leads to shock. In such cases there is always a gluten-induced potassium deficiency, often accompanied by magnesium and/or calcium deficiency.

6. Do you have strange or addictive reactions to alcohol?

   ❑ yes   ❑ no

   Either may also signal gluten sensitivity. We know that alcohol causes and aggravates a leaky gut; many authorities believe that a leaky gut is a common cause as well as a consequence of food allergies and gluten sensitivity.

7. Are you a smoker?

☐ yes ☐ no

A powerful tobacco addiction can also signal gluten sensitivity. Smoking can amount to a form of neurochemical "self-medication" for those who have problems with gluten. Smoking delays diagnosis and allows the progression of the disease. Such addictions are very difficult to break because quitting means more than simply dealing with the fleeting experience of withdrawal. It will bring about a reduction in general health and, in many former smokers, major depression—which will persist until the underlying problem with gluten is diagnosed and treated.

8. Do you struggle with anxiety and/or depression?

☐ yes ☐ no

These are common signs of gluten sensitivity.

9. What about your visual perceptions? Have you ever been sitting quietly, staring into the distance when things appeared much more distant than is possible? Or maybe they were distorted?

☐ yes ☐ no

If you have had such sensations, you may well have a problem with gluten.

10. What about your sleep habits? Do you usually have difficulty getting to sleep?

☐ yes ☐ no

11. Do you have an excessive need for sleep?

    ❑ yes ❑ no

12. Are you disoriented and confused when you awaken?

    ❑ yes ❑ no

13. Do you have to get up frequently during the night to urinate?

    ❑ yes ❑ no

14. Are you, or have you ever been, a bed wetter?

    ❑ yes ❑ no

    Such patterns suggest a problem with gluten, dairy proteins, or both

15. Do you often have difficulty finding the energy for life's daily demands?

    ❑ yes ❑ no

    Your body may be giving you an early warning. Lethargy of unknown cause is another common sign.

SHORT STATURE IS YET ANOTHER IMPORTANT SIGN OF A PROBLEM WITH GLUTEN

Several physical features, including your height and weight, can identify significant risk factors. People of below normal height, and especially children in the lowest 10th percentile, should, in the absence of a solid medical explanation for their stature, consider testing. Because susceptibility to the hazards of gluten is largely genetic, even where short stature appears to be a family trait, the possibility that gluten is an underlying cause in all family members should not be ignored.

Short stature and growth retardation can provide important warnings. Just as reduced stature was part of our ancestors' transition to agriculture, growth stunting continues to be a factor in celiac disease. In fact, half of all young celiacs over the age of two years are short compared to their peers.

There are many reports of short stature in connection with undiagnosed celiac disease. Some groups report rates of undiagnosed celiac disease in about one quarter of the subjects studied. Others report that as many as half of the individuals of short stature, when the cause of their short stature was unknown, have been diagnosed with celiac disease when tested. Little wonder that these researchers repeatedly urge testing all people of short stature for celiac disease. Even where growth hormone abnormalities are found, celiac testing is warranted because gluten can suppress growth hormone release.

OBESE CELIACS NO LONGER A CONTRADICTION

Obesity is another warning sign that gluten may be at the root of your difficulties. Despite the long-standing perception that celiac disease leads to frail, wasting, undernourished individuals, there are more obese and overweight celiacs than underweight. This is revealed through random testing for celiac disease.

MAKING USE OF REGULAR MEDICAL CHECKUPS

There are also a number of important warning signs that commonly show up in the routine lab tests done at the time of your annual medical checkup. These test results, when low-normal levels or deficiencies are indicated, will alert and benefit those with a high index of suspicion of celiac disease and gluten sensitivity.

Even when blood values approach the boundary of the normal range, those that should be carefully checked include:

- iron deficiency and iron deficiency anemia
- folate deficiency
- elevated free homocysteine
- vitamin B_{12} deficiency
- elevated or high-normal serum alkaline phosphatase often associated with gluten-caused bone loss (interestingly, zinc deficiency, often found in celiac disease, is commonly associated with low-normal alkaline phosphatase)
- chronically elevated liver enzymes of unknown cause
- low or low-normal serum albumin

If you suffer from chronic iron deficiency or iron deficiency anemia, or if regular iron supplementation just keeps your results at the low end of the normal range, there is cause for concern. The part of the small intestine where most iron is absorbed is the same part of the intestine where, in celiac disease, the greatest damage is often caused by gluten. Hence, iron deficiency anemia of unknown cause should routinely lead to testing for problems with gluten.

Folate is a B vitamin that is critical to neurological development and maintenance and is often depleted among those with untreated celiac disease. In order to prevent spina bifida, folic acid supplementation is of prime importance to women wishing to become pregnant. Low folate levels should alert us and should encourage appropriate testing.

An excellent predictor of risk for heart attacks and strokes is the level of free homocysteine in your blood. It may be elevated in as many as 30 percent of all people with a history of heart attacks. As with cholesterol and blood-pressure measurements, routine testing for homocysteine should be part of your annual physical. When it is high-normal or elevated, this is cause for concern. The good news is that these levels indicate deficiencies of folate, vitamin B_6, and/or vitamin B_{12}, which can often be remedied by supplementing a high-potency B complex. It may also be an indication of underlying celiac disease, known to cause such deficiencies. When one's homocysteine does not respond well to B vitamin supplementation, gluten sensitivity should be considered as a cause. For people with such deficiencies, a strict gluten-free diet might be just what the doctor ordered.

YOUR MEDICAL HISTORY

In addition to monitoring your routine test results, examination of your medical history can also be very revealing.

Low Blood Pressure

Chronically low blood pressure, defined as a systolic pressure of under 90 and a diastolic of less than 60, is also common among celiacs and should signal concern if your medical records reveal such a history. All too often, this is touted as a sign of good health when it actually may indicate a serious problem with gluten. Low blood pressure is usually accompanied by an inclination to fainting and sensations of light-headedness. A significant minority of celiacs will also demonstrate elevated blood pressure, so absence of low blood pressure should not be taken as a means of ruling out celiac disease.

Heartburn, Esophageal Reflux

If your history reveals that you have repeatedly been given medications for heartburn, or today what is fashionably called esophageal reflux, there may be cause to suspect celiac diesease. Similarly, if you are one of the many Americans who frequently consume over-the-counter antacids, testing for celiac disease may be very helpful.

Vitamins C and K, Bleeding and Bruising

Some researchers believe that the condition of vitamin C deficiency—scurvy—is common among children with celiac disease and can result in bleeding in the bowel or under the skin, or both. Vitamin K deficiency can also cause a wide variety of bleeding problems and may be the cause of some of the cases of intestinal hemorrhaging or bleeding following dental surgery that have been reported in people with celiac disease. Patches of red or purple rash are found in about 10 percent of newly diagnosed celiacs and may be the result of either of the above deficiencies or an autoimmune disease where there is a deficiency of blood platelets.

Looking for Mineral Deficiencies

Despite ample intake of dietary minerals, some people with undetected gluten sensitivity suffer from multiple deficiencies. Because of the inflammatory erosion of the intestinal lining, they are not absorbing these minerals well. Their bones become weaker, they grow very slowly, they perform poorly in school, they are more likely to become anemic, they heal more slowly, they begin to complain of chronic pain syndromes, and/or their immune systems fail to protect them from recurring infections. One common denominator with all of these conditions may be a lack of adequate iron, zinc, magnesium, selenium, and/or calcium for proper immune function. In the absence of trauma or dangerous infection, these people may often appear healthy.

Coughing, Wheezing, Shortness of Breath, and Gluten

A wide range of lung problems, including chronic bronchitis and asthma, characterized by chronic wheezing, coughing, shortness of breath, or difficulty in breathing, are commonly caused or made worse by gluten. Researchers are reporting that one-third of celiac patients have respiratory allergies. From a variety of allergic lung conditions, to defects in the lining of airways, to ulcers on the lung walls, to diffuse bleeding in the lungs and chronic obstructive pulmonary disease, gluten-related problems abound in asthma. Poor breathing from lack of adequate oxygen exchange is often the result. Lung disorders found in association with celiac disease sometimes show, on biopsy, evidence of a mucosal defect in the lungs that is similar in appearance to that found in the intestines. Therefore, chronic lung disease should also signal concerns about an underlying problem with gluten. We recommend that anyone with respiratory allergies get tested for gluten sensitivity.

Other Signs from Your Medical History

If you have struggled with repeated bouts of multiple, very painful sores inside your mouth, called aphthous ulcers or canker sores; if your fifth fingers are short and palms orange; if your fingertips are clubbed; if your fingernails are thin, brittle, and spoon-shaped; or if your nail beds remain pale when compressed, any of these can signal the presence of celiac disease or gluten sensitivity.

ARE YOU A MEMBER OF A HIGH-RISK GROUP?

Your medical history will also include specific ailments and diseases. Such conditions can warn of gluten sensitivity even when they appear to be unrelated. There are several general categories of illness where gluten sensitivity should be considered. They are:

- allergies
- autoimmunity
- bowel disease
- cancer
- growth retardation
- learning disorders

- lung disease
- psychiatric ailments
- reproductive problems
- seizures

High-Risk Candidates for Celiac Disease— Are You One of Them?

1. All first-degree family members of those with non-celiac gluten sensitivity or celiac disease. Some now argue for testing second-degree relatives.
2. All insulin-dependent diabetic (IDDM) patients and all first-degree relatives of these patients.
3. All autoimmune thyroid patients (both underactive and over-active) and all first-degree relatives.
4. All patients with chronic neurological or neuromuscular conditions of unknown cause (e.g., ataxia and peripheral neuropathies).
5. All patients with chronic liver disease/abnormally elevated liver enzymes of unknown cause. This includes primary biliary sclerosis, the disease that recently resulted in the premature death of NFL football legend Walter Payton.
6. All osteoporotic children (e.g., children suffering from frequent or easy/low impact bone fractures).
7. All postmenopausal osteoporotic women unresponsive to conventional therapies.
8. All epileptics with histories of migraines, ADHD, and/or calcium deposits in brain tissue.
9. All individuals suffering from chronic severe headaches unresponsive to conventional medical intervention, especially those with associated complaints of dizziness or imbalance.

continued

10. All patients with iron deficiency or iron deficiency anemia of unknown cause.
11. All pregnant women, especially those with a history of infertility, miscarriage, low birth weights, anemia, or other unfavorable pregnancy outcomes.
12. All children being considered for a diagnosis of ADHD.
13. All children with learning disorders.
14. All CD patients supposedly on a strict gluten-free diet, but with persistent or recurring symptoms.
15. All patients with Down syndrome.
16. All people with Turner's syndrome.
17. All people with major depression unresponsive to conventional antidepressant medication.

Your Work History

Your line of work, past and present, can also be an important factor in determining your risk of gluten sensitivity. Among flour mill and bakery workers, researchers have found dramatic increases in IgG class antibodies against gluten, the same antibodies that form from eating gluten. Their findings suggest that people working with flour are more likely to develop a systemic immune response to gluten through a reaction in the mucus that lines the lungs.

Your Family Tree

When examining your family health history, the presence of any of the ailments that are found more commonly in celiac or gluten-sensitive patients should also alert you to the possibility of your own increased risk of celiac.

Dr. Chris Reading and Ross Meillon of Australia have provided an ex-

Family History of Celiac Disease, Eight Years of Chronic Diarrhea, and Finally a Diagnosis . . .

The day I received my celiac diagnosis, I cried. After eight years of steadily increasing diarrhea, I finally had the answer. I had been through so many tests. I initially blamed my ailments on drinking some bad water when visiting my sister in Texas shortly after my second child was born in 1991. I had mentioned several times to my family doctor that my father had celiac disease, but it wasn't until November 1999 that I asked to be tested for celiac. I was diagnosed after an endoscopy and biopsy.

I also cried that day because I was sad. My father got so sick he died at age sixty-six from complications of celiac disease. He didn't have the resources we have today. He was handed a small book of recipes from the Hospital for Sick Children, Toronto, Canada. He researched in the library, I am sure, but he missed out on the wonderful connections of the Internet.

I often wonder if the lack of nutrients in my body caused me to contract breast cancer at age thirty-seven. All of my doctors said there was no connection, but I saw my father go through chemotherapy when he ended up having lymphoma. I often wonder if they are just not sure. My tears flow so easily anymore. I was feeling so abnormal and so sick—I can understand fully why people turn to antidepressants with this condition. I have found the silver lining to this black cloud and am living a fuller life now.

Lynn P.

cellent guide for developing an informative chart of your family's health history in their book *Your Family Tree Connection*. There is plenty of evidence to support such an approach. Almost half of the close relatives of celiac patients have increased intestinal permeability and, hence, a greater likelihood of both gluten sensitivity and celiac disease. Cancer also strikes family members of the celiac patient more often than others.

By beginning to think about disease susceptibility in light of one's family and, hence, genetic background, a wide range of preventive strategies becomes an active part of one's life. For instance, if a woman has given birth to a child with spina bifida, there is a clear case of folate deficiency and, hence, an increased risk of celiac disease in the mother. Further, one out of every fourteen patients with Down syndrome has undetected celiac disease. If you have a child with Down syndrome or a child with spina bifida, testing for gluten sensitivity and celiac disease is the next logical step.

If you are a member of one of the groups of people who have an unusually high risk of having or developing celiac disease, you absolutely should be routinely tested for both gluten sensitivity and celiac disease. Due to concern about latent celiac disease, if the initial blood screening is negative, you should schedule to be tested again every few years.

The patterns of information drawn from these five areas of your life and your family history offer a clear sense of whether you should seek testing for gluten sensitivity and celiac disease. The next chapter offers information about the wide variety and relative value of these tests.

Testing for Gluten Sensitivity
in All Its Forms

Now that you have a sense of what your risk might be, you will want to choose a test or series of tests appropriate to your risk, concerns, and budget. This is an issue that appears simple enough, but it is a little more complicated than that. There are several important mistaken beliefs about celiac disease that should be corrected. For instance, we have heard from individuals who were being investigated for celiac disease, but they were already on a gluten-free diet. With one important exception—a rectal challenge—there is no diagnostic procedure yet known that will reliably identify celiac disease after the patient has been following a strict gluten-free diet for just a few weeks. Sometimes testing is unreliable after only a few days. This chapter offers information that explains the various tests that can address your unique needs, and it will guide you past the many pitfalls of testing.

WHAT ARE YOU LOOKING FOR?

There are a variety of tests that will identify gluten sensitivity or celiac disease. Some tests will identify one condition while suggesting the other, while other tests will only identify or suggest one form of gluten problem. From a wide range of blood tests; to skin, rectal, and intestinal biopsies; to genetic testing; to saliva testing, our responses to gluten can be tracked in a number of ways. Each form of testing has its own unique strengths and weaknesses. Each offers important insights into how we react to gluten, so your choices should be shaped by your individual needs and test availability.

Issues of cost, convenience, and comfort may also be important in making the right selection. Because we are all unique and each of us reacts in a slightly different manner, it is not satisfactory to rely on a single form of testing. Your choice should be based on your unique needs and circumstances, not your doctor's convenience or level of knowledge. For instance, people whose siblings have been diagnosed with celiac disease might choose testing to determine if they have the genetic HLA markers for celiac disease or gluten sensitivity. A negative test will tell them all they need to know—that they have little risk of ever developing a problem with gluten. A positive test, on the other hand, will often indicate that this particular family member either has, or may soon have, an identifiable problem with gluten.

IMPORTANT ANSWERS TO BE FOUND IN HLA-DQ GENETIC MARKERS

Since genetic testing of your white blood cells is becoming increasingly available, you and your family may wish to make use of this important blood test to determine your inherited propensity to develop gluten sensitivity and/or celiac disease.

Dr. Kenneth Fine, a world-class researcher in this area, recently stated that HLA-DQ2 and/or HLA-DQ8 is present in about 43 percent of the normal American population. Dr. Fine believes that if one has such a genetic predisposition for developing a gluten-induced disease, the wisest approach is to avoid this disease-causing food.

In some cases, however, genetic testing may have little value. Those with non-autoimmune thyroid disease, for instance, have about the same risk of showing these genetic markers as any member of the general population. Such a person would benefit more from examining their risk factors, as outlined in the previous chapter, to determine whether there is any need to be concerned about gluten. If there is cause for concern, a more specific test should be chosen.

SMALL INTESTINAL BIOPSY

One individual contacted us reporting that she had been reassured that it takes four to six months for gluten-induced intestinal damage to heal, so a biopsy will identify celiac disease for up to six months after beginning a gluten-free diet. While it is true that it can take that long or longer for gluten-induced injuries to completely heal, it is a mistake to believe that a biopsy can produce an accurate diagnosis when consuming a gluten-free diet.

The biopsy is simply a sample of the cells in the intestinal wall. These cells are completely replaced every few days. This rapid replacement lends itself to extremely rapid healing of the very region that is being examined for injuries that are signs of celiac disease. In many cases, the intestine will appear perfectly normal after just a week or two of strict compliance with a gluten-free diet.

Everyone with a healthy intestine has millions of fingerlike projections on their intestinal wall called "villi." They improve the absorptive efficiency of the intestine by increasing the surface area through which nutrients can be absorbed. The flattening of all villi would reduce this surface area to a fraction of that of a healthy intestine. Such a reduction of surface area will cause a substantial failure to absorb nutrients from the food that passes through the intestine.

The current test that is touted as the "gold standard" for the diagnosis of celiac disease is a biopsy, taken by endoscopy. It is a process where a tube is passed down the throat, through the stomach, and into the small intestine. Tiny tissue samples are then taken from the intestinal wall for examination under a microscope. If the biopsy shows a flat surface, and a gluten-free diet shows in improvement on a second biopsy, then celiac disease is diagnosed.

This procedure was once without much controversy. When only those with a flat intestinal wall were considered candidates for a diagnosis of celiac disease, this disease was thought to be rare.

But this is not accurate because of the range of damage that can signal celiac disease. Dr. Michael N. Marsh has devised an ingenious system for categorizing the stages of gluten-induced damage to the intestinal wall. It not only offers a standardized approach to evaluating intestinal biopsies for the diagnosis of celiac disease but also encourages a fuller understanding of the immune mechanisms at work in celiac disease.

The Marsh system aids diagnosis of immune reactions to gluten that result in a range of damage to the intestinal wall. Because celiac disease is so variable, a more dynamic system for reading biopsies was necessary. Celiac symptoms wax and wane, and damage to the intestinal wall varies from one location to the next, and with the passage of time. The Marsh system has captured the range of intestinal damage that can result from celiac disease in a simple way that allows pathologists to uniformly identify the presence or absence of this disease. With the exception of Type 0, which depicts healthy tissue, from Type 1, indicating an infiltration of immune cells called intraepithelial lymphocytes, to Type 4, indicating tissue damage that is very resistant to treatment, each category of tissue damage indicates a level of intestinal injury that is commonly found in celiac disease. Celiac disease may thus be identified at an earlier stage and from biopsies that would previously have been viewed as inconclusive.

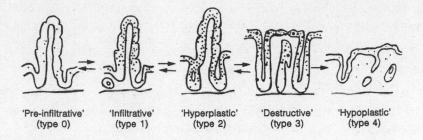

'Pre-infiltrative'	'Infiltrative'	'Hyperplastic'	'Destructive'	'Hypoplastic'
(type 0)	(type 1)	(type 2)	(type 3)	(type 4)

If you envision the inside of the intestine as the area above each of the biopsy samples depicted above, you can see that less surface area is available for nutrient absorption, as the gluten-induced damage progresses. Type 3 and 4 lesions are quite flat.

There is currently considerable variation in perspectives, from one pathologist to the next, regarding the signs that suggest the possibility of celiac disease. Some pathologists have insisted that their job is simply to describe the microscopic appearance of these tissues without ever suggesting the possibility of celiac disease. The Marsh system removes this problem by providing a set of templates for evaluating biopsies and providing clear guidelines and criteria for when to consider celiac disease.

In the past, the gastroenterologist or endoscopist often relied on the pathologist to raise the question of celiac disease, and the pathologist awaited the suggestion of celiac disease from the gastroenterologist. Despite clear signs, it was often never mentioned. Little wonder celiac disease was so rarely diagnosed! Thanks to the Marsh system and other advances in diagnostic testing, the number of such errors should diminish.

GLUTEN CHALLENGE

A gluten challenge is the process of consuming multiple daily servings of gluten-rich foods—as is common in the average Western diet—in order to gauge the body's reaction. Breakfast, for example, would likely include toast or cereal. Snacks might be cookies, crackers, muffins, or pastries. Lunch might contain sandwich bread or pizza, and the evening meal might include pasta, piecrust, or Yorkshire pudding, along with a flour-thickened gravy.

The major pitfall of such a gluten challenge is that it is often undertaken by those who have been following a gluten-free diet as the result of their own research or on the advice of a health-care practitioner or friend. Whether motivated by the difficulty of the gluten-free diet, concerns for family members, issues related to insurance coverage, income tax considerations, or other factors, such individuals later want laboratory or biopsy confirmation from a doctor for the diagnosis of celiac disease. But, if a patient has already begun a gluten-free diet and the intestinal wall has thus been given a chance to heal, it can take as much as five years or more after returning to eating gluten before the intestinal damage characteristic of celiac disease will show up on a biopsy. It is often too late to obtain a biopsy-based diagnosis except through a rectal challenge, which is discussed later.

SUGAR-ABSORPTION TEST FOR LEAKY GUT

The sugar-absorption test does not diagnose any disease. It is often used to identify increased intestinal permeability, or "leaky gut." The test is based on recognition of the complex interactions between several indigestible sugars called "disaccharides" and the function of different parts of the gastrointestinal tract. We are unable to metabolize these sugars, so whatever we absorb into our blood will be excreted in our urine. In a healthy person, after swallowing measured amounts of the sugars— lactulose and mannitol—insignificant quantities of them should be absorbed into the bloodstream.

Because molecules of each of these sugars have different properties, even where there is inappropriate intestinal leakage, more of one sugar will be absorbed and pass into the urine unchanged, thus identifying the leaky gut, along with the location of its greatest permeability.

Even the most vocal advocates of this test are unlikely to see it as a definitive test when used in isolation. However, it is a valuable adjunct to other testing. For instance, this test can make a second intestinal biopsy unnecessary for confirming a celiac diagnosis. Reduced intestinal leakage, after about a month on a gluten-free diet, will confirm the diagnosis. It is also a valuable companion to screening blood tests, providing a clearer picture of the condition of the intestine.

The sugar-absorption test is limited to identifying relative improvements. The improved state in one patient may still exceed the degree of leakiness found in an untreated celiac patient. It is also limited by another factor. Alcohol consumption, antibiotics, steroids, nonsteroidal antiinflammatory drugs, many non-gluten food allergens, spices, hormonal variations, infections, injuries, surgeries, and many conventional cancer therapies can alter intestinal permeability very rapidly. The sugar absorption test is designed to identify only a current state of increased intestinal permeability. Results of this testing can therefore be quite misleading, as there are so many other factors in addition to celiac disease that are not controlled in the context of this testing that can exert a substantial influence on the test results.

BLOOD TESTING

The reliance on intestinal biopsies may soon be a thing of the past. Extremely specific and reproducible blood testing is poised to take its place. Some of these blood tests offer the added advantage of identifying people who are mounting an immune response, regardless of intestinal damage. Other tests will only identify advanced celiac disease. There is quite a range of tests, offering considerable choice to health-care consumers. The development of blood tests that can identify the antibodies relevant to gluten sensitivity may well be one of the greatest scientific leaps of the last century.

Anti-Gliadin Antibody (AGA) Blood Test

If you put gluten in a petri dish with human internal organs, the gluten damages these tissues. If a gluten-sensitive individual consumes gluten, he or she runs the risk of damaging organs and tissues throughout the body. Therefore, finding out if gluten is getting into your bloodstream and creating havoc makes good sense. Now, recall that gliadin is an important but very troublesome member of the family of gluten proteins. Testing for antibodies produced and directed against gliadin is currently one of the best ways to determine whether gluten is getting into our blood and, hence, if we are in danger.

Our immune systems can't tell the difference between a gluten protein and another foreign protein that is a structural part of bacteria or a virus, so we react the same way against all foreign proteins, by developing specific antibodies against these proteins. Two classes of antibodies that are sensitized to gliadin are sought in antibody testing. These classes are identified as IgG and IgA antibodies.

Importance of Testing for IgG and IgA Anti-Gliadin Antibodies and IgG Antibody

The most common criticism of AGA blood tests is that they are not specific enough. Elevated levels of gliadin antibodies are found in many people with a variety of ailments, many of which do not include celiac disease. They are even found in apparently healthy people. Because of this, such abnormal AGA results are often dismissed as meaningless. The IgG class of antibodies is by far the largest group of antibodies in the human body. These antibodies don't identify any specific disease and are often found elevated in people who have few or no symptoms. And they do last a long time, especially compared with other classes of selective antibodies. A comparatively brief period when there is leakage of gluten into the bloodstream could result in a positive AGA blood test for up to six months or so.

How, you may ask, is this test useful? It identifies a leaky gut. Unlike the sugar-absorption test, it identifies any relatively recent event of significantly increased intestinal permeability when gluten proteins were leaked into the bloodstream.

IgG is a test that also warns of the likelihood of additional delayed-onset food allergies and the possibility of toxic-liver overload. It may also point

Gluten Sensitive and Food Allergic— Diagnosed with Blood Tests

I developed a concave area on my back at about the level of my kidney. It was slowly growing in size and had become very painful. Our family doctor suggested that it was some kind of fatty tissue necrosis. I visited three different specialists. Each of them admitted that they were unable to offer a treatment that would reverse or halt the disease. They could not even identify it. I was given pain medications. I slept through the night, and much of the day. I gained weight from my inactivity. I was depressed and barely able to look after my two children, who were six and eight years old at the time.

Because the doctors were stumped, I had blood drawn and sent off for testing for celiac disease. I had elevated gliadin antibodies. Our doctor was skeptical about the value of these tests.

I then had blood drawn for IgG ELISA testing, which revealed sensitivity to gluten, dairy, and seventeen other foods. Within a week of eliminating the identified offending foods, the pain disappeared. I discontinued the pain medications and needed less sleep. The following week, the concavity became itchy. The afflicted area began to shrink.

Even now, if I accidentally eat gluten or dairy, I develop joint pains.

Kari K.

to the source, or a contributing factor, in a current disease state. More important, it signifies that an individual has become sensitized to gliadin and is at risk of gluten sensitivity or any of the forms of celiac disease.

All patients with elevated IgG and/or IgA antigliadin antibodies should be treated seriously and monitored carefully. All such individuals should be routinely blood tested for celiac disease.

IgA Antibody

Another class of gliadin antibody that is easily identified, and often quite useful, is the IgA antibody. It is usually much shorter lived than the IgG antibody. This makes it very useful for monitoring dietary compliance. However, it is also valuable, especially in combination with IgG antibody testing, for screening large groups when looking for celiac disease. These anti-gliadin antibody blood tests are comparatively inexpensive, and when used together they are quite good at identifying those who should be biopsied and tested for endomysium antibodies.

Endomysium Antibody (EMA) Testing

Endomysium is connective tissue that sheaths certain muscle fibers. The development of the endomysium antibody test resulted from recognition that antibodies against this tissue are present in more than 90 percent of celiacs who are consuming gluten, yet they disappear quite rapidly after excluding gluten. This form of blood testing was developed following recognition of the connection with celiac disease and demonstrates that celiac disease is an autoimmune condition since these antibodies attack endomysium.

We have heard from patients who have had blood drawn for endomysium antibody testing for celiac disease while consuming a gluten-free diet. Let us stop and consider this for a moment. While it is true that IgG anti-gliadin antibodies will survive for six months or longer, endomysium antibody tests are often used to check whether celiac patients are following a gluten-free diet. If the endomysium antibodies are low or unde-tectable, the celiac patient is thought to be following the diet. How much sense can it make to test for antibodies to identify celiac disease when the patient is already following a gluten-free diet? This mistake can be terri-bly misleading and can have disastrous consequences.

This test is very sensitive, and it will identify 90 percent or more of those patients with flat intestinal walls, but some evidence suggests that it is less reliable for identifying cases with milder intestinal damage. Some warn that reliance on blood testing alone will lead to missing a significant number of cases of celiac disease. Perhaps, but there are some larger issues to consider. Without this blood test, currently we would not be aware of the startling frequency with which this disease is silently present in the general population. Even granting that some cases will be missed by this screening, when carefully conducted, endomysium antibodies are reveal-ing a rate of celiac disease that is very close to 1 percent of the American population.

When used in conjunction with IgG and IgA anti-gliadin antibody testing, valuable information can be offered, thus allowing the patient to make an informed choice about whether to continue to consume gluten.

The shift toward a heavy reliance on anti-gliadin antibody and EMA blood tests has been under way in Europe for over a decade. It certainly offers a huge improvement over the current situation, where only a tiny fraction of celiac disease is ever diagnosed. Although a less than perfect solution, it does offer some exciting possibilities, and as part of the grow-ing arsenal of weapons against dietary gluten, we heartily endorse its use when limited to case finding. However, a negative EMA blood test has limited value for excluding celiac disease. This test is also limited by the need for individual observation and evaluation of stained blood cells.

Tissue Transglutaminase (tTG) Antibody Testing

In the field of blood testing for celiac disease, the tissue transglutami-nase (tTG) test is currently the newest entity. It is another step toward solving the puzzle of celiac disease. Transglutaminase is an enzyme that forms a normal part of endomysium and is involved in tissue repair. It is the part of endomysium that anti-endomysium antibodies attack. Since tTG antibodies can be identified by computer, it eliminates one of the greatest weaknesses of EMA testing mentioned in the preceding paragraph.

The tTG test usually identifies about 98 percent of those who have celiac disease, and it is a very specific test that can be used to rule out celiac disease in about 95 percent of cases. This test appears to be superior to endomysium antibody testing, not only because it is less costly but also because it is a little better at identifying celiac disease and because interpretive bias is reduced by the use of computer scanning.

A New Development in the Offing

A tremendously convenient level of testing for celiac disease may soon be available on the basis of this new development. A simple finger stick and blood blot is all that is required for this new test, and results can be available within an hour. It is expected to be commercially available in the United States prior to the publication of this book.

RECTAL CHALLENGE

There is another exciting innovation for the diagnosis of celiac disease that offers an answer to many of the current problems and testing errors. A twentieth-century medical researcher who arrived in the twenty-first century well ahead of most of us, Michael N. Marsh, M.D., has initiated new directions in celiac research for this millennium. In addition to creating the standard by which well-informed pathologists throughout the world evaluate intestinal biopsy samples for signs of celiac disease, Marsh and his colleagues have also developed a test that is superior to the intestinal biopsy for identifying celiac disease. Known as a rectal challenge, it is a procedure that can be conducted in the doctor's office using plastic instruments, and clear, quantified results can be available in a matter of hours.

As the name suggests, it is a procedure that first involves taking a biopsy of the rectal mucosa. Then gluten slurry is placed into the biopsy site, followed by a second biopsy from the same area four or more hours later. Computer analysis of these tissue samples identifies immune reactions to gluten if they are present, thus leading to a diagnosis of celiac disease. While our description is somewhat oversimplified, the critical issue is that this test differentiates those whose immune systems are sensitized to gluten from those who do not react to it.

When the rectal challenge was first introduced in the late 1980s, it was not well received. The most common objection was that it identifies too many people as having celiac disease. Many authorities considered it impossible that so many people could have this disease.

Since that time, innovative blood-testing methods such as EMA tests and IgG, IgA, and tTG ELISA tests have dramatically increased the rate at which celiac disease was diagnosed to the point where it is now found in about 1 percent of the general population when it is sought. In ELISA blood testing, a scanner is used to identify molecular complexes attacked by endomysium antibodies and can be used to gauge the reaction of a range of antibodies to gluten and to detect many food allergies. Therefore, the most common objection to the rectal challenge is therefore not a legitimate one, as shown by the growing use of blood tests.

The second most common statement of resistance to this test is the embarrassing nature of the entire procedure. The AGA, EMA, and tTG ELISA tests are certainly more comfortable, convenient, and less invasive. We can only acknowledge this criticism of the rectal challenge as valid and recognize that this will deter many from seeking this test. The EMA and tTG offer accurate, reproducible lab results but, when negative, do not completely rule out gluten sensitivity or celiac disease. For those individuals with stout hearts and a willingness to undergo this procedure, it can be very valuable.

Rectal Challenge Advantage

1. Unlike the intestinal biopsy, it identifies an immune reaction to gluten and only gluten.
2. It costs much less than a biopsy.
3. It is a little more embarrassing but a lot less invasive than the biopsy.
4. It reduces the risk of error-related patchy intestinal lesions.
5. It will not miss the milder cases of celiac disease that are missed by blood testing alone.
6. It will reliably identify celiac disease for a full six months after beginning a gluten-free diet, unlike any other test for celiac disease.
7. The biopsies are analyzed by means of a computer. This eliminates the risk of human error due to variations in perception from one person to the next, which is a problem in some types of blood tests, as seen in jejunal biopsies and EMA.
8. The results are reported in a single numerical form, so their interpretation is infinitely less subjective and lend themselves to standardization.
9. Patients can receive their test results much more rapidly, usually by the following day, although that will soon be overshadowed by the speed with which tTG test results can be made available.
10. There is a reduced risk of complications due to the test. Although they are extremely rare in jejunal biopsies, the risk is even smaller when taking a rectal biopsy, especially since only one day's procedure is necessary for a firm diagnosis. This added safety is especially important for infants, pregnant women, the elderly, and the gravely ill.

SKIN BIOPSY, DERMATITIS HERPETIFORMIS, AND IgA DERMATOSIS

Dermatitis herpetiformis, a gluten-induced, extremely itchy, blistering rash, has only recently been recognized as a subset of celiac disease, although the debate of this issue appears to be subsiding. This offers another approach to obtaining an accurate diagnosis of celiac disease. If you suffer from the gluten-induced skin lesions that are called either Duhring's disease or dermatitis herpetiformis, a simple skin biopsy taken from uninvolved skin can provide a solid diagnosis. Most dermatologists will be able to take a biopsy and send it for evaluation. The biopsy will reveal an irregular layer of IgA deposited just below the basement membrane of the skin. This will confirm the diagnosis of dermatitis herpetiformis and, by implication, celiac disease.

Differentiation between dermatitis herpetiformis linear IgA dermatosis has, until very recently, been the only challenge. The pathologist could confidently identify dermatitis herpetiformis where the microscopic view of a layer of IgA antibodies, deposited just under the skin, was quite rough and irregular. In linear IgA dermatosis, on the other hand, the layer is quite regular and smooth in appearance.

In June 2001, however, one group of researchers reported a case of linear IgA dermatosis in a patient who was also diagnosed with celiac disease. The skin disease, along with the associated celiac disease, responded to a gluten-free diet and returned on gluten challenge. We would like to see a variety of skin diseases similarly investigated.

GENETIC TESTING

If you or your family members have a genetic susceptibility to celiac disease, it can now be easily identified. Commercial blood tests are increasingly being used to identify genetic markers on white blood cells, such as

HLA-DQ2, HLA-DQ8, and HLA-B8, all of which are found more frequently in those with celiac disease than in the general population. The argument can legitimately be made that a greater number of people with these genetic markers do not have and will never develop celiac disease. However, it is reasonable and prudent to use such markers as guides to suggest the possibility of celiac disease, thus raising the level of suspicion for celiac disease for these individuals while significantly reducing the number of individuals who turn out to have negative biopsies.

DIAGNOSIS AND LIFELONG GLUTEN-FREE DIET

The process leading to a diagnosis of gluten sensitivity, celiac disease, or dermatitis herpetiformis is often very trying. The testing choices we make will also shape how we deal with the results. We recommend strict compliance with a gluten-free diet for everyone who tests positive for any of the diagnostic tests, as well as for those close relatives of celiac patients who have the genetic markers for celiac disease. We also recommend several other forms of testing and careful monitoring for additional illnesses. The next chapter explains the diet and important follow-up testing.

Life After Gluten

Finally, you have a diagnosis—one you can use to improve or rebuild your life. Regardless of the gluten-induced health hazards you wish to avoid or the health problems you want to correct, the starting place is a gluten-free diet. If you're new at this, you will quickly find that a gluten-free diet is not just a case of eliminating bread, breakfast cereals, and pasta. Gluten grains and the countless foods and recipes made from them permeate and shape our entire culture. The comfort they provide has caused some of their widespread seductive, almost sensual appeal, which also makes them difficult to give up. Throughout this chapter we provide information about how to reduce the stress of the transition to a gluten-free lifestyle.

Adoption of a gluten-free lifestyle offers many rewards to those who are willing to meet this important challenge.

DEALING WITH PHYSICAL ADDICTION TO GLUTEN

The addictive nature of gluten is often overlooked. For some, the first days and weeks of following a gluten-free diet are characterized by food cravings, disorientation, irritability, sleepiness, depression, mental fogginess, fatigue, and/or shortness of breath. If you are a member of this group, the very fact that you are experiencing many of these symptoms should reinforce the need to exclude gluten from your diet. These are common symptoms of withdrawal or detoxification from gluten-derived opioids and brain neurochemical imbalances. The evidence suggests that about 70 percent of celiac patients will experience these symptoms when beginning a strict gluten-free diet.

We have stressed the need, when a gluten-free diet is indicated, for strict avoidance of all traces of gluten. There are several good reasons for this strident recommendation. Ask anyone who has managed to break an addiction and they will likely tell you that one of the secrets of their success is that they haven't "cheated" with small amounts on special occasions or at a weak moment. Such cheating actually keeps the addiction alive or restarts it. The previously addicted ex-smoker and the alcoholic ex-drinker will often state that they are one cigarette or one drink away from starting their addiction again. They are often quite vigilant about that first, apparently minor, slip because it is the one that begins their slippery slide back into addictive behavior.

Most individuals who have celiac disease or non-celiac gluten sensitivity are also addicted to gluten. The morphine-like peptides from gluten frequently stay intact because the bonds between some sequences of amino acids are quite resistant to digestion. Those who have a leaky gut will allow these opioids and other large peptides to enter the bloodstream. The addictive process has probably been at work in most gluten-sensitive and celiac individuals for many years, probably since childhood. This makes elimination of gluten a great deal more challenging than might be expected. It certainly requires more than a halfhearted suggestion from a family doctor or gastroenterologist.

INFORMED AFTERCARE

Counseling

The counseling that was too often recommended as the only response to legitimate symptoms of gluten sensitivity and celiac disease may now have some value. As with any other addiction, its successful resolution will often require a systematic, well-considered approach. Many support groups provide the necessary contact with others who have gone through the same experiences, or some people may require the intervention of addictionology health professionals who are versed in the treatment of addictions.

Dietary exclusion of gluten not only involves battling the physical and psychological facets of this experience but also requires coming to terms with the socially excluding nature of this diet. Few social occasions do not include food and drink. Where gluten-free alternatives exist, the risk of contamination is quite large. Even the beverages must be considered with caution. This often decrees social isolation and a reluctant avoidance of all social functions by the gluten sensitive.

Another important problem arises when gluten sensitivity is trivialized. Gluten-sensitive and celiac patients need to be given the necessary support and guidance for breaking their addiction. They also need to be carefully monitored. Where appropriate, most will also need to be tested and treated for the health problems that developed as a result of their prior gluten-consuming lifestyle.

Join a Celiac Support Group

We urge you to join a support group. Fortunately, there are many hundreds of them, with more sprouting up around the world every day. Take a moment to visit the Internet to search for support groups in your area.

Support groups usually produce informative newsletters that provide information on sources and identities of gluten-free foods, product safety, how to stay truly gluten-free, and ingredient changes by particular manufacturers. The social events provide opportunities for members to share experiences, recipes, and new information on a wide range of topics that are relevant to those pursuing a gluten-free lifestyle. The counseling provided by the more seasoned members can sometimes be invaluable to the newcomers, and the shared sense of community can be valuable to all.

A Gluten-Free Household

If you have a newly diagnosed celiac in your family, there are several good reasons to implement a gluten-free household. First and foremost, gluten sensitivity and celiac disease run in the family. Not only will it certainly be a safer environment for the celiac/gluten-sensitive individual, but it will also help other family members develop a better understanding of the challenges faced by the gluten-sensitive family member. And it will ensure an improved diet for the entire household, which may lead to some unforeseen health improvements for other family members. A gluten-free environment can also reduce the workload for the family cook by allowing the preparation of a single meal for all.

Testing for Additional Food Allergies

Additional food allergies are the rule among the gluten sensitive. Testing for common food allergies such as milk, soy, and eggs is a critical part of the program for regaining health after identification of a problem with gluten. IgG ELISA blood testing for delayed food allergies is our current recommendation.

Bone-Density Testing

Seventy percent of all undetected celiacs have significant bone loss. That being the case, bone-density testing should be conducted annually.

This will ensure that the diet and appropriate supplementary bone nutrients are effectively reversing the damage previously done by gluten. This regular testing is particularly important because of the current preoccupation with calcium supplementation at high doses for those with compromised bone-mineral density. To date, the published research that shows the most promise for remineralizing bones in celiac patients—beyond simply following a strict gluten-free diet—clearly favors magnesium and zinc, as well as vitamins D and K supplementation.

Regular Thyroid Testing

Laboratory testing for thyroid function is usually limited to blood tests that look closely at the thyroid-stimulating hormone (TSH) and free T4. Under usual circumstances, this is perfectly appropriate. However, given the high rate of autoimmune thyroid disease among the gluten-sensitive, more extensive testing is warranted in any gluten-sensitive individual and his or her immediate family members. Regular testing should also include monitoring blood levels of triiodothyronine and thyroxine (T3) along with anti-thyroid antibodies to ensure that any gluten-induced autoimmune thyroid problems are identified early. Early detection and a subsequent gluten-free diet have been reported to reverse autoimmune thyroid disease.

Glucose-Tolerance Testing

Appropriate testing should also be conducted in response to the risk of hyperglycemia (high blood sugar) and Type I diabetes, which is substantial among those who are gluten sensitive. First-degree family members of known gluten-sensitive individuals should also be monitored for Type I diabetes along with celiac disease.

Liver-Function Testing

Liver function should also be watched carefully in the gluten sensitive. Some liver enzymes will often be quite abnormal at the time of diagnosis. In many cases, this will soon normalize on a gluten-free diet. We believe it is important to be aware of this inclination if you are one of the gluten-sensitive individuals whose liver reacts abnormally to gluten. Such insights probably do not warrant a gluten challenge, so testing liver enzyme levels at the time of, or shortly after, diagnosis will provide valuable information.

Quarterly Eye Exams During the First Year

It may sound excessive to recommend such frequent eye exams, but the headaches and discomfort caused by blurred vision are often quite disruptive to one's life. Since many newly diagnosed celiacs experience quite a lot of change during the first year or so, these checkups and consequent modifications of correction may help reduce the negative impact of the changes and difficulties.

Dental Work

It is important to let your dentist know about your sensitivity to gluten, because it can cause enamel defects such as horizontal and vertical grooves, as well as an increased frequency of dental caries. In addition, chronic periodontal disease with unhealthy gums could possibly be the result of your gluten sensitivity—not the result of poor oral hygiene, as is often assumed. The gluten-free diet will often reverse this problem, so minor interventions coupled with a "wait and see" approach may be preferable to surgical interventions in gum disease associated with gluten sensitivity.

NUTRITIONAL CAUTIONS

Once you are aware that you are gluten sensitive, it is also important to avoid certain pitfalls.

Desensitization Therapies

These procedures can be an effective means of reducing symptoms of gluten sensitivity, celiac disease, and other allergies. Administering small amounts of an allergic or toxic substance in an attempt to desensitize a sensitized individual is the principle by which allergy shots work. They may also work on the principle of adaptation that was described by Hans Selye seventy years ago. However, such therapies, especially in the area of powerful genetic predilections, as found in gluten sensitivity, risk the very consequences that Selye also identified in his work so long ago. Early death was the consistent result of adaptation to chronic physical stressors. Premature death is the consequence of continued exposure to gluten in the gluten sensitive.

In essence, desensitization therapies disarm the warning system provided by your body. By reacting to a given substance, your body is letting you know, either with symptoms or with abnormal immune responses, that this substance is not healthful. We suspect that such reactions have developed through the evolutionary process. If foods or other substances make us feel ill, and if we know which foods these are, we should—unless the addictive cravings exceed self-discipline—avoid them. Those who do not feel ill in response to allergic substances in their environment are more likely to succumb to the harmful effects of these allergens. Thwarting this efficient, finely tuned system that warns us to avoid allergenic foods is inappropriate.

Trace Quantities of Gluten

For the same reasons, taking a cavalier attitude toward consumption of trace quantities of gluten can also prove to be hazardous. Regular ingestion of small amounts may create an adaptation to gluten that is similar to that created by desensitization therapies. Through chronic ingestion of trace quantities, a psychological perspective may develop. Given the addictive nature of gluten, maintenance of a mostly gluten-free diet risks either a chronic and unpleasant battle with addiction or the beginning of a slippery slide back to regular gluten consumption.

Gluten Ingredients in Pharmaceutical Products

Recall that less than one gram of gluten daily is enough to perpetuate a diseased intestinal lining. With this in mind, it should no longer seem a petty issue that non-medicinal food ingredients in pills from the pharmacy can pose quite a challenge, especially for those who are acutely sensitive to gluten.

Many pharmaceutical companies have contracts with food suppliers for starch-binding materials. Unless explicitly instructed otherwise, the contractor will understandably choose the least expensive supplies. Sometimes that will mean that corn starch will be used. At other times, wheat starch will be most cost efficient. The net result is that, unless a pharmaceutical manufacturer has specified the source of the starch binder in its contract with the food supplier, you may be exposed daily to sensitizing doses of gluten when taking your medication. Your pharmacist, doctor, and manufacturer may not be able to say whether there are trace amounts of gluten in the non-medical ingredients used to fill your prescription. The best strategy is to ask your doctor to specify that the prescription is open to substitution from a manufacturer that uses gluten-free binders. Many do.

Steroids

Steroid medications, although valuable in certain instances, may pose several important hazards to those who are gluten sensitive. Demineralization or thinning of our bones is already a major risk as the result of years of gluten consumption. Steroid medications add to that risk as a consequence of further worsening of a leaky gut, complicating blood-sugar regulation and demineralizing our bones. Many gluten-sensitive individuals have spent years battling intestinal, vaginal, and systemic fungal infections as a direct consequence of steroid medications.

With the exception of steroids needed to stabilize breathing in an asthma attack, we urge extreme caution in the use of these drugs by those who are gluten sensitive.

Dapsone

Although this leprosy medication is quite effective for reducing the extreme itching associated with dermatitis herpetiformis lesions, high doses have been shown to cause cancer in rats. Given the extraordinary increased risk of cancers, the frequency of neurological disease, and the overlap of the latter conditions among those with gluten sensitivity or celiac disease, considerable caution seems in order. The best and safest therapy for dermatitis herpetiformis remains strict avoidance of gluten.

OPTIMAL NUTRITION ON A GLUTEN-FREE DIET

Following a gluten-free diet is not at all easy. Because it is a difficult diet for most people to follow, it is especially challenging for the first six months or so while you adjust your thinking, increase your knowledge, and develop the shopping and eating habits needed to be strictly gluten free.

In general, a gluten-free diet excludes all foods made from wheat, rye, and barley. This prohibition includes avoidance of pastas, pancakes, batters, breads, and other baked foods, except where they are prepared with flours made from rice, corn, nuts, amaranth, quinoa, and other gluten-free foods. Appendix B provides a complete listing of unsafe sources of flour, but there are a few important issues that need explanation.

Strict avoidance of gluten quickly leads to healing of the small intestinal lining and improved nutrient absorption. This can have some surprising implications that require cautious implementation of the best dietary practices. In today's high-pressure world of tight time lines and fast food, it is no small task to consistently eat a healthy, well-rounded diet. In general, we recommend that, wherever possible, meals should consist of a wide variety of fresh meat, internal organs, poultry, fish, fruit, vegetables, and antioxidant herbs and spices.

Eat whole, unprocessed, and organically grown food when possible. Like unprocessed foods, organically grown food has fewer man-made chemicals and toxic metals, and often has a higher nutrient content, including improved protein quality and up to 30 percent more vitamin C, iron, magnesium, and phosphorus.

We also recommend five to nine servings of a wide variety of non-allergenic fruits and vegetables each day. The more vegetables and fruits one eats each day, the less likely he will develop food allergies and intolerances. Such healthy eating habits will reduce inflammatory disease and result in fewer heart attacks, strokes, and cancers, and overall better health.

A healthy diet of fruits and vegetables should include one bountiful, mixed salad daily with extra-virgin olive oil, flaxseed oil, or an essential fatty acid oil blend. Quercetin-rich foods such as apples, red and yellow onions, chives, and all kinds of berries are strongly recommended. Also, be sure to include the many excellent detoxifying cruciferous vegetables such as broccoli, cauliflower, brussel sprouts, kale, cabbage, watercress, kohlrabi, and bok choy.

In addition to a daily broad-spectrum multi-vitamin/mineral, we recommend that you supplement with extra vitamin C and natural, mixed vitamin E and carotenoids. Frequent use of antioxidant, anti-inflammatory culinary spices such as fresh garlic, ginger, and turmeric (Indian curry), as well as herbs such as oregano, dill, thyme, and sage in your food preparations is also extremely valuable.

Fats and Oils

Repeated high-temperature heating of oils and fats converts them to pro-inflammatory, cancer-causing substances, so fried foods need to be strictly avoided. Lower-temperature steaming, boiling, broiling, stir-frying, and roasting are preferable to frying. It is particularly important to avoid all hydrogenated fats, oils, and margarines. The evidence indicates that when eaten in excess, these man-made oils, found in many processed foods, behave as pro-inflammatory, carcinogenic substances in our bodies.

Be cautious about pursuing a low-cholesterol diet. Extremely low-serum cholesterol (under 160 mg/dL) is associated with an increased risk of strokes, cancer, sudden death, and suicide. Instead of following such a diet, we recommend that you increase your consumption of a blend of essential fatty acids every day. These include liberal amounts of omega-3 fatty acids (fish oil, flaxseed oil, and walnut oil, e.g.), omega-9 fatty acid (extra-virgin olive oil), and a more limited intake of omega-6 oils (vegetable and seed oils) and arachidonic acid (animal fat), including the yolk from boiled and poached eggs.

Animal Protein

Eat four- to six-ounce servings of fresh, unbreaded, unfried, oily, non allergenic fish two to five times a week (salmon, Alaskan halibut, orange roughy, sardines, Chilean sea bass, trout, and mackerel, e.g.). Large fish such as shark and swordfish are reported to contain high concentrations of mercury and should therefore be avoided. Weekly servings of shellfish, such as shrimp, crab, and lobster, can be very beneficial. Yet, you should be aware that shellfish are common allergens and may also accumulate pollutants.

We suggest eating lean red meat, boiled or poached eggs fortified with vitamin E and omega-3 oils, and omega-3 oil–rich wild game such as deer, elk, buffalo, and/or rabbit once or twice a week. In addition to being free of antibiotics and growth hormones, these meats add another important element to the diet by broadening the range of dietary proteins. Wild duck, goose, pheasant, and quail also provide many of the same advantages, including variety. Domestic poultry is also a healthful option when it has been range-fed and has not been treated with growth hormones and antibiotics.

Internal animal organs such as liver, heart, pancreas, and bone marrow should be part of our weekly diet as well. For hundreds of thousands of years our ancestors ate not only an abundance of wild game, fish, and shellfish when available but also appear to have preferred internal organs to muscle meat when the luxury presented itself.

Caution about Substituting for Gluten

It is important to establish eating habits that will ensure you get the greatest possible benefits from your gluten-free, allergen-free diet. For instance, gluten-free substitutes for treats such as cakes, cookies, pastries, and breads are much more calorie-dense than their gluten-containing counterparts. Underweight, newly diagnosed individuals who are in the habit of consuming large quantities of food may now be at risk of excessive weight gain because their absorptive capacities have increased dramatically, and these substitutes are so much richer in empty calories, causing abnormal spikes in blood insulin and sugar levels.

Newly diagnosed teenagers are particularly at risk for this increase in blood-sugar levels. The conventional adolescent diet in our culture is laden with foods such as rice, corn, potatoes, refined sugars, gluten-free snacks, and soda. Although these foods are gluten free, habitual over-indulgence elevates blood insulin and sugar abnormally, often resulting in obesity, high blood pressure, elevated blood fats, non-insulin dependent diabetes, and heart disease.

Additional Food Sensitivities

There are frequent reports of celiac patients continuing to suffer from chronic symptoms while following a strict gluten-free diet. Milk, soy, corn, egg, and other delayed-onset food sensitivities are commonplace among celiac and gluten-sensitive patients. With the elimination of offending foods, many lingering symptoms improve or disappear.

Remember that those who are gluten sensitive are also likely to have multiple delayed-onset food allergies, with dairy products heading the list along with corn, soy, eggs, citrus fruits, and seafood. Peanuts and/or yeast are also common allergens. IgG ELISA allergy testing is an important laboratory tool for identifying these hidden allergens and subsequently developing a healthy diet. Once allergic foods have been properly identified, a two- to four-day rotation diet should be planned. A wide variety of non-allergenic foods will help build a healthier body.

Beverages

Alcoholic beverages should be avoided during the first three to six months of healing. Alcohol causes or worsens a leaky gut, thereby perpetuating illness and delaying recovery. Also, in addition to eliminating soda from your diet, we recommend that you do not exceed two cups of decaffeinated or regular coffee each day. Consider replacing coffee with green or black tea. It is important to drink eight to twelve glasses of filtered water daily (roughly one ounce of water for every two pounds of body weight). Avoid tap and well water, if possible. Be cautious about substituting fruit juice for water or fresh whole fruits. Reports of weight gain and retardation of vertical growth in children have been reported.

Other Recommendations

Consume foods and beverages that are high in the anti-allergy, anti-inflammatory, antioxidant bioflavonoid quercetin; these include apples, green and black teas (but not coffee), red and yellow onions (but not white onions), and red wine (but not white wine or beer). High quercetin dietary intake reduces the risk of premature death from all common causes.

A Day in the Life of the Gluten Free

You may want further clarification regarding how you can structure each day's gluten-free meals. Here is an illustrative example of such a diet, excluding allergenic foods on an individual basis:

BREAKFAST

*a cut of lean meat and/or 1 to 2 boiled or poached eggs fortified with extra
    vitamin E and omega-3 oils*
fresh fruit
a slice of gluten-free toast or a rice cake with jam
a cup of tea

LUNCH

mixed vegetable soup made with plenty of bones
    or
Fresh steamed, broiled, or baked fish
    or
shellfish with a bountiful mixed salad, vegetables, and a fresh-fruit cup

EVENING MEAL

poultry, organ meat, or muscle meat
*a small amount of carbohydrate such as potatoes, whole-grain rice, or gluten-
    free pasta*
steamed or raw mix of vegetables

SNACKS

celery or carrot sticks
pickles
pickled herring
olives
nuts and seeds

OCCASIONAL TREATS THAT HAVE A VERY HIGH GLYCEMIC INDEX
    (caution is required)

popcorn
corn or taco chips
potato chips
french fries
gluten-free rice cake, cookies, pastries, etc.
sesame snaps

The Rotation Diet

Eating favorite foods every day, even eating from the same food group day after day, is a recipe for developing food allergies. This is especially true for those who are gluten sensitive because of their propensity for a leaky gut. When the gut is leaky, a certain amount of food protein will be absorbed into the bloodstream. If this occurs daily, or several times a day, the immune system is bound to become sensitized to it and begin to mount an immune response to it. Remember, it is the foreign proteins in microbes that your immune system recognizes and reacts to. Any foreign proteins, including those from foods that arrive in the bloodstream in any quantity, are likely to spark an immune response. That likelihood increases with daily or more frequent exposure.

We recommend that after eating a particular food, you avoid that food group for two days. This is called rotating your foods, or a rotation diet.

If you eat potatoes on Monday, for instance, you should avoid that food until Thursday. It can be a bit of a chore to keep track of all these food issues, but the benefits will soon encourage your continuation of a rotation diet. One important tool for following a rotation diet is a food diary. Just as you might keep a daily appointment book, you would simply record all the foods you eat each day.

Rotation not only reduces the risk of developing further food allergies but also forces you to eat a wider variety of unprocessed, unpackaged, less chemically laden foods, which is also an important strategy for achieving optimal health. The food diary reinforces such healthy eating habits.

Eating Gluten-Free Away from Home

As with the person who carries cards that provide a convenient means of making contact to conduct business, you may wish to carry a card that provides appropriate information to restaurant employees. Restaurant cards can be printed in the same format as a business card. An example of such a card is provided below:

I NEED YOUR HELP. I BECOME VERY SICK WHEN I EAT GLUTEN GRAINS.
Hence, I follow a gluten-free diet. I need to avoid all forms of wheat, rye, oats, barley, triticale, spelt, and kamut. This includes all malt, TVP, TPP, HVP, HPP, and MSG. Unless it is clear that they do *not* come from one of the above grains, I must also avoid all vegetable starch, food starch, and natural flavors.

Thank you for your assistance and cooperation.

Our experience with restaurants has been very positive. We find that most are quite happy to help and are usually quite successful in preparing gluten-free meals.

DIETARY SUPPLEMENTS

Some fats are absolutely essential to humans. We cannot maintain good health without them, yet our bodies are unable to synthesize them. Cereals are very low in omega-3 essential fatty acids. Substituting other cereals for gluten grains is a step in the right direction, but this approach continues to displace dietary meat and other sources of omega-3 fatty acids and further compromises one's nutritional well-being. We must get these fats from our diets or supplements.

Eight amino acids are equally essential to human health and must come from our food supply. Some essential vitamins are abundantly available in animal products, such as vitamin B_{12}, yet they are not found in other food sources, including gluten cereals. We humans are members of a very select animal group. Guinea pigs and humans are the only mammals that cannot synthesize their own vitamin C. Hence we are also the only animals at risk of developing scurvy. Cereal grains contain very little of this health-promoting vitamin. By displacing fruits and vegetables, the consumption of cereals reduces our vitamin C intake.

All of these factors combine to counter the current high complex carbohydrate, high dietary gluten-grain fad. Our cells can utilize carbohydrates for energy, but they can also use fats. The difference is that there are some fats that we must get in our diet (called essential fatty acids) while there are no known essential carbohydrates.

A properly prepared animal protein–dominated, low-cereal diet that includes plenty of fruits, vegetables, nuts, and seeds offers us the nutrients essential to our good health. Failure to absorb these nutrients, and the absence of other critical nutrients from these cereal-derived foods, has created many of the nutritional deficiencies that plague our culture, despite our calorie-rich lifestyles.

Nutrient absorption is so variable, even in treated celiacs, that individual assessment, leading to individually tailored advice, is the best approach. Depending on which part of the intestine is injured, the extent of the damage, how often accidental ingestion occurs (for instance, those who do a lot of traveling would be at greater risk), and how long the damage persists, there can be quite a variation in need for a particular supplement. Although a complicated issue, supplementation is very important to achieving optimal health; therefore, gluten-sensitive individuals should pay considerable attention to this important issue. Regular monitoring of blood levels of vitamins and minerals is an important first step. During the first year, monthly or bimonthly monitoring offers a means of checking for deficiencies, as well as monitoring the impact of supplementation.

Magnesium Supplementation

Magnesium is essential for proper maintenance of the parathyroid gland. Not only is this gland a major regulating factor in your body's calcium metabolism, but endomysium antibodies have also been shown to cross-react with the tissues of this gland. That means that many individuals with celiac disease will derive important benefits from magnesium supplementation. We can only speculate that similar benefits might be derived by many of those who are gluten sensitive. Magnesium deficiency may play a key role in many of the common symptoms and medical conditions overrepresented in untreated celiacs and gluten-sensitive individuals, including osteoporosis, migraine headaches, muscle pain or spasms, major depression, chronic fatigue, premenstrual syndrome, asthma, autism, heart disease (cardiomyopathies) in children, and seizures.

Magnesium supplementation over a two-year period results in a raised serum parathyroid hormone and improved bone density.

The impact of magnesium supplementation is an excellent example of the need to tailor recommendations to the gluten sensitive on an individual basis. Based on clinical improvements, there can be little doubt that gluten-sensitive individuals are almost universally deficient in this important mineral. However, magnesium levels are very difficult to measure accurately, so it is probably more useful to monitor the many functions that improve as a result of magnesium supplementation. For instance, improvements in bone density and parathyroid hormone levels in the blood can both be good indicators that magnesium supplements are providing benefits. Reduction or disappearance of bone pains, muscle twitching, and an inclination to muscle cramping can all indicate the value of supplementing magnesium.

This important mineral also loosens the bowels. This can be a real blessing for those gluten-sensitive individuals who struggle with constipation, but it requires caution and careful attention from those who are inclined to diarrhea.

Calcium Supplementation

Calcium supplements are taken by individuals who are unable to get enough calcium in their regular diet or who have a need for more calcium, such as growing children, postmenopausal women, the elderly, pregnant or breast-feeding women, and many celiacs. Supplements are used to prevent or treat several conditions that may cause hypocalcemia (not enough calcium in the blood). The body needs calcium to make strong bones. Calcium is also needed for the heart, muscles, and nervous system to work properly. Given almost universal bone mineral depletion in adult-diagnosed celiacs, calcium supplements are extremely likely to be recommended. We remind the reader that bone health and density depend on multiple factors and nutrients, including but not limited to magnesium, zinc, boron, vitamin D, and vitamin K, in addition to calcium.

However, excessive calcium supplementation at the expense or avoidance of other key bone nutrients can lead to several problems for those who are gluten sensitive. High intakes of calcium supplements may interfere with the absorption of other nutrients such as iron and zinc. Intake of calcium supplements may also interfere with the absorption of concurrently consumed medications, and vice versa. Other potential adverse effects of chronic intakes of high doses of calcium include milk-alkali syndrome (ectopic calcium deposition) and hypervitaminosis (i.e., in the case of supplements containing calcium and vitamin D).

Further, calcium and magnesium share the same transport mechanism for absorption across the intestinal barrier. Excessive calcium supplementation may overwhelm this mechanism, inhibiting the absorption of magnesium, thereby aggravating a preexisting magnesium deficiency or inducing a magnesium deficiency where it might not otherwise occur. Magnesium has also been identified as a common cause of osteoporosis in celiacs, even on a gluten-free diet. Some researchers have found evidence for a ratio of 1:1 in hunter-gatherer diets, suggesting a similar ratio for supplementation of calcium and magnesium.

Selenium Supplementation

Selenium is a mineral that is used to treat some skin diseases, and small-quantity supplementation has been shown to reduce the risk of some cancers. Selenium deficiency is common in non-celiac gluten-sensitive patients and untreated celiacs. Selenium deficiency continues to be one of the conditions commonly overrepresented in the gluten sensitive, leading to the risk of developing many other conditions such as proneness to esophageal and other cancers, heart disease in the form of cardiomyopathy, infertility, miscarriages, kidney disease, chronic liver disease, asthma, underactive thyroid, testosterone deficiency (selenium is required for production of both thyroid and testosterone hormones), Down syndrome, autism, and accelerated death from AIDS (selenium deficiency increases the death rate from AIDS by twentyfold!). Given the increased risk of cancer and premature death among the gluten sensitive, selenium supplementation can be used to counter both the limitations imposed by malabsorption and poor diets alone and the limitations caused by selenium depletion in the soil of some farming regions.

Iron Supplementation—A Word of Caution

There can be little doubt that iron deficiency is an important, widespread problem in gluten sensitivity. Often, simply by eliminating gluten from the diet, the problem is solved. On the other hand, additional iron as an iron supplement can be very important for establishing and maintaining optimal health in those with persistent iron deficiency. It is extremely important to identify iron deficiency early in an infant and young child's life because chronic iron deficiency is thought to be associated with permanent loss in intelligence, school performance, and other cognitive abilities. Be aware also that vitamin B_{12} deficiency coexists in about 15 percent of children with iron deficiency and that cow's milk allergy is another extremely common cause of blood-loss iron deficiency in children. All these factors have to be monitored and effectively treated.

Common symptoms of iron deficiency may include pale complexion, pale fingernail beds, rapid heartbeat, chronic fatigue, easy bruising, excessive nose bleeds (this may also indicate a vitamin K deficiency, commonly found in celiacs), diminished exercise endurance or tolerance, indigestion, difficulty swallowing, loss of taste, symptoms of "restless leg syndrome" (creepy, crawly sensations in legs, relieved by movement of the legs—magnesium is helpful here, too), heartburn, chest pain, anxiety or depression, and attention and/or learning deficits in children.

Be aware that you don't want to supplement with iron unless you need it. Excess iron can pose a hazard to men, postmenopausal women, those who frequently eat red meat, and those who regularly supplement with large doses of vitamin C (over 500 to 1,000 mg daily). Iron supplementation should be managed in collaboration with your doctor on the basis of regular blood tests that have confirmed existing iron deficiency.

To repeat, do not take iron supplements unless you need them. Excessive iron can cause potentially life-threatening damage to the heart, liver, and pancreas.

Potassium Supplementation

Potassium deficiency is associated with irregular heartbeat, salt-sensitive high blood pressure, enlarged kidneys, kidney failure, recurring kidney stones, and fatal strokes. Commonly, chronic diarrhea is the underlying cause. Therefore, potassium is another mineral that should be closely monitored. Normally, a gluten-free diet with lots of fresh fruits, vegetables, lean meat, fish, and poultry will supply you with all the potassium you need. On occasion the diet proves inadequate in supplying potassium, and supplementation should be considered after collaboration with your doctor. Potassium deficiency, in association with muscle wasting, weakness, and paralysis, has been reported in celiac disease.

One note of importance: Magnesium and potassium deficiencies often coexist in celiac disease. If you have persistently low serum potassium levels, not corrected with proper diet or supplementation, more magnesium supplementation is frequently needed. If low magnesium and potassium levels coexist, magnesium supplementation will often bring both the magnesium and potassium levels back to normal values.

B Vitamin Supplementation

B vitamin deficiencies are common in gluten-sensitive individuals and those with celiac disease. Folate, B_{12}, and B_6 deficiencies are of special importance due to their relationship with neural tube defects in newborns, seizure activity, and increased risk of heart attacks, strokes, and cancer associated with elevated blood levels of homocysteine. Vitamin B_6 deficiency has also been reported to play a role in carpal tunnel syndrome, major depression with fatigue, asthma, PMS, attention deficit disorder, and the nausea and vomiting experienced during pregnancy.

When our absorptive capacity is compromised by gluten, it is difficult to predict which of these B vitamins, and in what quantity, we should supplement. Because we excrete any excess that we do not need, conventional wisdom suggests oversupplementation, trusting urinary excretion for maintenance of optimal levels.

We are aware of at least one report of nerve injury as the result of excessive vitamin B_6 supplementation in excess of 150 mg daily. We recommend exercising caution when supplementing with this B vitamin.

For those with chronically low blood pressure, a common feature of celiac disease, caution is also appropriate when supplementing with vitamin B_3. Some individuals choose to begin with very small doses.

Vitamin A Supplementation

Vitamin A deficiency is commonly associated with recurring infections, especially in children. Vitamin A deficiency is also the leading cause of blindness in children worldwide. The ability to safely take vaccinations also appears to be closely linked to vitamin A status. Deficiency of zinc and this vitamin may also play a key role in food allergies.

Although vitamin A deficiency is often a problem in gluten sensitivity, it is not safe to oversupplement. Excess vitamin A has been observed to cause headaches and dry skin. More critically, doses in excess of 10,000 IU daily may cause birth defects. Much higher sustained doses can have a devastating impact on your own health and, in rare instances, may be fatal.

Vitamin A supplementation should not be undertaken carelessly. Collaboration with your doctor and regular testing are critical parts of your program for supplementing with this vitamin if you show signs of deficiency.

Vitamin E Supplementation

Vitamin E deficiency, perhaps in conjunction with selenium deficiency, may be associated with accelerated heart disease, strokes, Alzheimer's disease, Parkinson's disease, diabetes, cataracts, and prostate cancer. One or more of the fat-soluble vitamins, vitamin E included, have been reported to be deficient in celiacs. However, caution is also important in taking vitamin E supplementation. These vitamins are stored in body fat, and toxic accumulations may occur.

Vitamin D Supplementation

Vitamin D deficiency is thought to be a causative factor in osteoporosis, osteomalacia, psychological depression, suicide, and colon cancer. Low blood and tissue levels have been reported in untreated celiacs.

The safest, cheapest source of this vitamin is exposure to sunlight. However, with mounting concerns about skin cancer, this source of vitamin D has lost some of its appeal. Those institutionalized in hospitals and nursing homes, those living at more northerly latitudes, and those who work long hours inside are even less likely to get adequate vitamin D from the sun. Vitamin D supplementation has now become the norm.

DIETARY DANGERS

Oats: To Eat or Not to Eat, That Is the Question

The inclusion of gluten-containing oats remains a bit of a hot topic among those who follow a gluten-free diet. Oats advocates point to current studies showing no change in shape or size of the intestinal villi of celiac patients. Since the gliadin proteins that cause damage to the intestinal villi have been identified and are not present in oats, oat advocates consider them safe to include in the gluten-free diet. Many also argue for including oats because they believe that it will provide a valuable substitute for some of the missing foods made from wheat, rye, and barley, thus making the diet more tolerable.

Conversely, those who wish to see oats continue to be excluded from a gluten-free diet argue that, because oats are handled with the same farm machinery and stored and milled in the same facilities as the other three gliadin-rich grains, gliadin contamination is inevitable.

Further, while it is true that the proteins that cause villous atrophy are not present in oats, opponents argue that all other gluten proteins in this grain have not been proven harmless. In fact, glutenin, another gluten protein, is currently receiving a lot of attention in the research community as the protein associated with asthma and autoimmune skin conditions.

Oats also cause abnormal changes to white blood cells inside a test tube, and, most important, many celiacs develop symptoms in response to oats. This may result from immune responses that cause increased intestinal permeability or other negative health consequences.

We have already established that there are many more cases of non-celiac gluten sensitivity where there is a leaky gut in the absence of villous atrophy than cases of celiac disease. It is not yet clear whether any of the gliadin proteins identified as causing damage to the villi are also causing intestinal permeability in the non-celiac gluten sensitive. If the same proteins are simply causing a different form of damage to the intestinal wall, the distinction between gluten sensitivity and celiac disease becomes even more blurred. If there are non-gliadin proteins in gluten that cause a leaky gut in those who are gluten sensitive, they might also be causing increased intestinal permeability in celiac patients.

DON'T EAT OATS!

Given the evidence, we advocate excluding oats until there is clear evidence of its safety by demonstrating that all proteins from this grain do not cause either intestinal permeability or any other form of damage to the gastrointestinal tract or elsewhere.

Wheat Starch

There are thoughtful arguments on both sides of the wheat starch debate as well. When tested, celiacs consuming wheat starch as part of an otherwise gluten-free diet do not show intestinal damage or suggestive antibodies in the blood. Wheat starch advocates claim that since wheat starch is often tolerated by very sensitive celiacs, it is likely harmless, at least for those who do not react to it. In England, where the gluten free diet has been shown to reduce the risk of cancer and other sequels of untreated celiac disease, wheat starch has long been accepted as gluten free.

We hasten to point out that a failure to react or a lack of observable intestinal damage do not guarantee that gluten is not causing harm. Furthermore, given the rate of asymptomatic silent celiac disease, the use of symptoms as evidence of sensitivity is highly questionable when evaluating the safety of wheat starch. Intestinal biopsies also fall far short of that perfection when used to identify low levels of gluten consumption due, in part, to the frequency of patchy damage to the intestinal wall. This also applies to the blood tests for celiac disease, especially when performed as single tests on people who are consuming only small amounts of gluten. The exception to this rule may be when EMA and tTG celiac tests are combined—a 94 percent sensitivity has been reported for those consuming wheat starch.

DON'T EAT WHEAT STARCH!

To add to the wheat starch confusion, there are two current studies that provide evidence in support of opposing sides of the argument. We take the position that claims for the safety of certain foods should be based on firm evidence. The purification process that separates wheat starch from gluten protein is not a perfect one. In the absence of a preponderance of evidence to the contrary, we err on the side of caution by recommending against the consumption of wheat starch.

Additives

Developing the habit of relentlessly reading ingredients lists on labels is a critical part of successfully following a gluten-free diet. Rule of thumb: Any processed food is suspect. In addition to avoiding wheat, rye, barley, triticale, spelt, kamut, malt, and oats, it is also important to be on the alert for the acronyms that can spell trouble: HPP, HVP, MSG, TPP, and TVP

Acronyms That Might Spell "Hidden" Gluten

Fu—dried wheat gluten
HPP—hydrolyzed plant protein
HVP—hydrolyzed vegetable protein
MSG—monosodium glutamate
TPP—textured plant protein
TVP—textured vegetable protein

(see the box above, where we spell out the words from this alphabet soup). While these substances may not be refined from gluten, there is a good chance that is exactly where they come from. Vegetable starch, food starch, modified food starch, and natural flavors should also be avoided, as the source of these additives is difficult to determine.

There are good financial reasons that food manufacturers use these generic terms and acronyms to identify constituents of their products. This practice allows them to switch supply sources of these ingredients according to daily price changes or other market considerations, without the expense of changing their labels each time. Only when informed consumers pressure for changes in such practices will we see specific labeling with the full name of the ingredient on the label.

Other Hidden Hazards

Throughout the industrial world, laws governing food labeling allow manufacturers considerable latitude. The scientific reality is that trace quantities of gluten and other allergenic substances are difficult to identify. A United Nations commission operating under the auspices of the FAO and WHO sets the standards for food labeling and is called Codex Alimentarius. This commission has established minimum levels of gluten content that are allowed in foods labeled "gluten free." This may seem contradictory, even foolish, but it is a reality that has shaped labeling legislation throughout the world.

Closer examination reveals some reasonable arguments in favor of this perspective, if only because it is extremely difficult to identify and measure very small quantities of such gluten contamination, which would make more stringent legislation difficult or impossible to enforce. In many parts of Europe, where wheat starch has long been accepted as gluten free, this perspective may not raise eyebrows. However, the support groups in the United States, Canada, New Zealand, and Australia have long advocated a policy of zero tolerance.

At a recent international conference in Tampere, Finland, many visiting gluten-sensitive delegates from these zero gluten tolerance countries found themselves suddenly erupting with dermatitis herpetiformis lesions. This could have been the result of some other form of contamination, as they were presumably eating in restaurants most or all of the time. Conversely, it could have been the result of eating foods that contained wheat starch and oats, which form part of the "gluten-free" diet in these countries.

Due to the undeniably high prevalence of gluten sensitivity and the extraordinarily small amounts of gluten capable of mischief, we strongly encourage labeling that reflects the true nature of the contents of the food in question. If a food product is truly gluten free, we would want the labeling to reflect that. If, on the other hand, solid scientific evidence comes to light suggesting that some reduced level of gluten is permissible, we would expect the labeling to read something like "low gluten" or "gluten content does not exceed x parts per million." Then we will see the tens of millions of gluten-sensitive consumers placed in a much better position to make more informed, healthier decisions for themselves.

Common Sources of Contamination

If you live in a household where some residents are eating gluten, a shared toaster can be a source of difficulty. Sharing the same butter dish can also result in sharing a certain amount of gluten, perhaps enough to perpetuate sensitization.

When shopping, bulk bins can also be a source of contamination. Scoops from other bins, customers returning foods to the wrong bin, and inadequate cleaning of bins when store employees are switching bin contents can all result in problems. Although they are usually less expensive, we suggest avoiding foods sold in bulk bins.

It is also important to beware of gluten-free baking from a regular bakery. These products can be quite safe, but it is important to investigate first. If the bakery follows strict procedures to reduce the risk of contamination from contact with gluten-containing baked goods, you may be willing to take a chance on their products. We know of many gluten-sensitive individuals who fare very well on such products. Others have reported problems with such products.

Now that you are familiar with what it means to be gluten free, you can apply this knowledge to understand gluten's effect on many chronic illnesses. In the following chapters, we will reveal the role that gluten plays in many diseases and how a gluten-free diet can alleviate the ailments of many of these conditions.

The Cancer Connection

Cancer research throughout the last century offered great promise. The press heralded one exciting breakthrough after another, yet the cure and remission rates continue to be very disappointing. We believe we know part of the reason why.

Perhaps as a result of the requirements set by those providing research funds, or possibly because of the directions set by those who review research reports for publication, many cancer researchers have consistently looked in similar directions. Whatever the cause, when an individual or a group reported a hopeful finding, there was soon a stampede to similar research.

As a result of the massive body of research accrued during the war on cancer, we now know that

1. a wide range of genetic mutations can lead to cancer
2. almost everything in our environment can cause these genetic mutations

3. there are isolated areas of cancer treatment that actually do improve the quality of life and longevity for a minority of cancer patients

Despite the consistent failure of a majority of cancer therapies, there is often a quick dismissal of even mildly divergent perspectives, especially when they involve diet. It seems that many, at least in the realm of cancer treatment, have few answers but considerable disdain for the views of others. However, the scientific evidence simply does not support such a narrow view.

The avoidance of dietary intervention is confusing and disturbing. Many of today's mainstream cancer treatments sometimes cause horrible suffering to patients during the declining season of their lives, yet we have repeatedly heard the foolish assertion that a gluten-free diet will diminish the quality of the cancer patient's life. Purveyors of such nonsense should try following a gluten-free diet before uttering such thoughtless remarks.

WHAT ARE THE LIMITS OF OUR KNOWLEDGE OF CANCER?

Of course, if we had a full understanding of cancer, we would soon know the cure. Sadly, there is neither a complete understanding of cancer nor a reliable cure. For the most part, there are only contested theories and very debatable treatments, with a few rays of sunshine in an otherwise dismal scene.

There are at least two important ways in which our current knowledge of cancer is quite limited. We not only have an incomplete understanding of cancer—perhaps because of the narrow research focus dictated by economics and politically correct medicine—but we also have some mistaken ideas about the nature of the disease. It is the second limitation that poses the greatest problem. We often cling to many mistaken notions with an amazing tenacity. Perhaps desperation strengthens our grip, as cancer deaths continue at an alarming rate.

Historically, there are many examples of dearly held mistaken beliefs. Childbed fever, an infection transmitted by medical personnel, was once blamed on its victims. Pellagra, a deadly disease of nutritional deficiency, was once considered an infectious plague. The history of science is riddled with examples of such mistaken beliefs, which slow and misdirect research. To avoid this, until we can honestly claim significant cure rates, we should remain open to additional information and alternative perspectives. It is the absence of openness that limits the massive health-care and research industries concerned with understanding and treating cancer.

Many current cancer treatments are crude, cruel, costly, and often deadly. Cancer research proceeds at a dead-slow pace. While we await the very gradual expansion of knowledge about cancer, we must work with the evidence we have.

LET'S LOOK AT WHAT WE DO KNOW

We already know that cancers are very rare or nonexistent in primitive cultures consuming hunter-gatherer diets. We also know that where wheat and its near relatives are cultivated, we see the gradual emergence of cancer.

For instance, increased cancer risk among female farmers in Norway maps a clear connection between exposure to wheat and cancer, although the researchers reporting this connection blame the molds that grow on wheat for these cancers. In the United States, a correlation between wheat cultivation acreage and cancer deaths has been reported, although this increase was attributed to pesticide use. Other studies have suggested that whole-grain consumption will increase the risk of developing prostate cancer. Although the researchers consistently blamed other features of grain cultivation, there is a clear connection between the amount of grain that is grown and rates of cancer. Despite the popular belief that grains prevent colorectal cancer, some studies have shown that consumption of refined flours actually increases the risk of colorectal cancer.

In a report of children following a gluten-free, dairy-free, low-residue diet following conventional cancer treatments, there were huge reductions in the rate of enteritis, a condition that often results from abdominal radiation and chemical therapies for cancers. In this study, the rate dropped from 70 percent to zero. Not a single case of enteritis developed among those patients who followed this diet! Enteritis, with its associated infections and malnutrition, is frequently the cause of death in such cancer patients, so it is difficult to exaggerate the importance of this study.

In cases where celiac disease has been identified at the same time as cancer, there have been a few cases reported where a change in diet, in addition to conventional treatments, resulted in full remission of the cancer. In one case, a gluten-free diet certainly led to the disappearance of enlarged lymph glands that may have signaled lymphoma. Yet another patient with celiac-associated lymphoma improved when the only therapy was a gluten-free diet in combination with nutritional supplements.

There have also been reports in the peer-reviewed literature of cancer patients in the grips of apparently hopelessly fatal cancers who have experienced dramatic improvements and recoveries on a ketogenic diet. This diet provides energy through fats, not carbohydrates. Although this is a much stricter, more difficult diet to follow, it starves the cancer cells of the glucose they need to reproduce. It is the relentless reproduction of cancer cells and their displacement of healthy ones that is cancer's greatest threat. By slowing or halting this reproduction, the ketogenic diet allows the immune system a window of opportunity to battle these aberrant cells. Because this diet excludes gluten and can be dairy free, avoidance of opioids for pain management unleashes natural killer cells to attack the malignant ones.

This diet, originated in the 1920s, has recently received considerable public attention, as it can often control epileptic seizures when no known drug is effective. Part of the success of this diet in the treatment of such cases of epilepsy and cancer may also lie in its total exclusion of gluten.

Among those with celiac disease, the gluten-free diet has been shown to reduce the risk of developing cancer after about five years of strict dietary compliance. This is a group that otherwise has quite a large risk of developing any of a number of cancers, especially intestinal lymphomas.

This research, and a great deal of other evidence, points to the astounding possibility that our growing gluten gluttony is a major contributor to escalating cancer rates today. The evidence against gluten is certainly mounting. However, we leave the final judgment of that issue to future, more adventurous cancer research and to the reader.

HOW DOES GLUTEN INCREASE THE RISK OF CANCER?

There are certain peptides, or protein fragments, found in gluten and in casein, a protein found in milk, that look and act just like the narcotic known as morphine. They are hidden in an inactive state within the gluten and casein protein sequence, and are released by the digestive processes in the stomach and by pancreatic secretions. Once freed from the larger protein structure, they are highly resistant to enzyme digestion in the intestine. There is quite a large body of evidence establishing that these peptides found in gluten and dairy products may also be responsible for many of the health hazards associated with gluten. Some researchers have suggested that the opioids were the primary attraction for our ancestors who adopted agriculture. The physical, sensual comfort offered by the exorphins encouraged them to relinquish their healthier, less demanding hunter-gatherer lifestyles. Exorphins may be the determining feature of what we now call "comfort foods."

Gluten contains at least five distinct opioids—A4, A5, B4, B5, and C—and they are found repeatedly in the structures of a single protein. Gluten exorphin, A5, for instance, occurs at fifteen sites in a single glutenin protein. Although exorphins are less potent (0.5 mg of the most active of these exorphins are reported as about equal to 1nM of morphine) and variable in their strength, there can be little doubt that such a plentiful supply has helped shape the Western diet.

HOW EXORPHINS AID THE DEVELOPMENT OF CANCERS

It is an interesting paradox that, although the theory of cancer that we propose is not a mainstream perspective, it is built on a foundation of mainstream research. In later chapters, we examine some of the psychological impacts of gluten-derived exorphins, but for the moment our focus is on how these opioids aid in the development of various cancers.

Our immune systems have developed the ability to destroy damaged cells that might develop into cancer, but exorphins interfere with this defense mechanism. Natural killer cells are an important part of our immune systems that can act to identify and destroy cells with altered chromosomes—cells that might become cancerous. Natural killer cells have long been recognized as the body's first line of defense against many types of cancer. Once the cancer starts to spread, the function of natural killer cells is probably less important.

Opiates and opioids have repeatedly been shown to interfere with the action of natural killer cells. Whether these narcoticlike substances are used for pain management, to sustain addiction, or are unwittingly absorbed as partly digested proteins, they can all arrive in the bloodstream and inhibit our ability to ward off cancer.

There are two ways in which exorphins will act to deregulate natural killer cells. First, they can act directly on opioid receptors located on the natural killer cells, abolishing their protective function against cancer. In one report, this interference was shown to occur within thirty minutes of exposing blood from celiac patients to proteins from gluten. Second, they can act indirectly, through the part of the brain that controls the activation of natural killer cells, called the hypothalamic-pituitary-adrenal (HPA) axis. The evidence suggests that gluten and its fractions interfere with our immune systems' protective function in both ways.

CELIAC DISEASE AND ADDICTION

Because exorphins are biochemically similar to heroin, cocaine, and morphine, we should expect to see some similarities between untreated celiac patients and addicts. In fact, there are many similarities. Just as addicts experience powerful cravings, abnormal food cravings are commonly observed among gluten-sensitive and food-allergic sufferers, leading to the commonly used "food allergy–food addiction" diagnostic-descriptive label.

Addicts suffer the same compromised action of natural killer cells and are also at very high risk of developing certain cancers. There are many other ways in which the immune competence of celiac patients and addicts are similarly compromised. Thus, there are a number of ailments where celiacs and addicts share an increased risk. A close look at some of these overlapping risk areas may make this perspective clearer.

Let's look at the lungs first. Lung abscesses and cavities have been reported in celiac disease and opiate addiction. Pulmonary bleeding has also been reported in both celiac disease and addiction. Addicts and untreated celiacs also share a propensity for a variety of other lung disorders.

Another area of overlap is that both celiac patients and addicts demonstrate substantially higher rates of chromosome damage than the general population. The evidence suggests that both groups may be particularly slow at repairing cellular DNA, which may be a key element in the development of cancers.

The immune system abnormalities found in heroin and cocaine addiction, including enlargement of gastrointestinal lymph nodes, are sometimes confused with, and even misdiagnosed, as lymphoma. The lives of those addicted to narcotics are at risk through forms of urban violence that are obscure to most of us, with a life expectancy of about thirty years. Despite their short life expectancy, these individuals contract cancers at a dramatic rate. Heroin addicts have long been recognized as very susceptible to a variety of cancers. The heroin addict's risk of cancer is clearly not the result of advanced age. The increased risk is likely due, at least in part, to the action of opiates such as heroin and morphine on immune system function, especially natural killer cell function.

Celiac disease has been referred to as a premalignant condition, not only due to the very high rate of different cancers but also because of the symptoms it shares with lymphoma, including enlargement of gastrointestinal lymph nodes. It is usual for exorphins from gluten to be absorbed into the circulation of patients with untreated celiac disease. These exorphins have been implicated in the association between a variety of psychiatric ailments and celiac disease. Many of these celiac-associated conditions resolve on a gluten-free diet. And these opioids likely explain the dramatic rates of cancer suffered by untreated celiac patients.

As with heroin addicts, patients with untreated celiac disease have a much greater risk of developing a variety of cancers. It is not much of a leap to conclude that exorphins are interfering with natural killer cell activity in the same way that heroine interferes with natural killer cell activity among addicts.

There are many similarities between untreated celiacs and opiate addicts in impaired natural killer cell function, altered T-cell function, generally reduced immune function, and altered spleen function, another important element of the immune system.

The time asserted for full recovery of an addict's immune system after drug withdrawal is three to five years. It is more than a coincidence that during the first five years of dietary compliance, celiacs experience a declining risk of malignancy on a gluten-free diet, with the greatest number of deaths due to cancer during the first three of these years.

All of these points of convergence define the overlap between celiac disease and opiate addiction. The dietary opioids may also prepare us biochemically for opiate addiction. They teach our bodies an inordinate appreciation for the effect of opioids and, hence, for opiates.

HAZARDS OF OPIATE PAIN MANAGEMENT IN CANCER

The research showing that opiates interfere with immune function has led some investigators to raise some important questions about the use of morphine for pain control in cancer patients, suggesting a search for alternatives. This is an important issue that should at least be raised as part of obtaining informed consent prior to the use of opiates for cancer pain management.

COMPARING CANCER RATES IN CELIAC DISEASE

In untreated celiac patients, there is a hugely increased risk of many types of cancer. Small intestinal lymphomas are found up to one hundred times as frequently in celiac patients. They also experience about twelve times the risk of esophageal cancer and about ten times the risk of mouth and pharynx cancers compared to the general population. Breast cancer, in the families of celiac patients, is twice as common as in the general population.

Cancer Rates in the General Population

How does this relate to cancer in general? There is reason to suspect that others, many of whom are only gluten sensitive, also absorb the opioids from gluten in their intestines into their bloodstream. This evidence leads to the reasonable conclusion that much of the current explosion of cancer rates is tied, at least in part, to recent and continuing increases in gluten consumption.

Dairy proteins are probably also involved in the escalating cancer rates. There are eight distinct sequences of amino acids in a milk protein called casein that have also been discovered to have opioid function.

They are called "casomorphins," and are not as potent as those derived from gluten.

Recall that hunter-gatherers were apparently immune to cancer. For at least five hundred thousand years, these ancestors of ours, with rare exceptions, did not eat a diet that contained gluten. Dr. Reading's cancer patients benefited from a gluten-free diet while undergoing conventional cancer treatments, and Dr. Donaldson's pediatric patients who were otherwise at grave risk of developing enteritis have also given us cause to value a gluten-free diet in the context of cancer treatments.

MALABSORPTION

Among those who recognize the threat of cancer for those with celiac disease, it is commonly understood and accepted that diet and the essential nutrients found in foods play a critical role in the cause of many cancers. We have known for half a century that celiac disease is characterized by a malabsorbing, leaky gut. Celiac patients not only leak larger proteins, such as exorphins, into their circulation, but also fail to absorb many essential nutrients. This is usually thought to result from the reductions of absorptive surface area in the small intestine. However, this view fails to explain the broad variations in type and extent of nutrient deficiencies that are displayed by untreated celiac patients.

There are many reports of a wide range of such deficiencies, including deficiencies in the minerals calcium, magnesium, selenium, manganese, copper, iron, and zinc and deficiencies in vitamins C, D, A, E, K, and a wide range of B vitamins. And herein lies a serious difficulty in recognizing celiac disease. Deficiency in each of the vitamins and minerals listed above will produce a set of symptoms that can usually be distinguished from each other. For each deficiency, there is often a range of possible symptoms and sets of symptoms. Sometimes, the number of variations in symptoms for one deficiency can be quite surprising. When compounded by the interaction of several or many deficiencies, the range of signs and symptoms can be enormous and quite confusing.

INSULIN ABNORMALITIES

To further add to the confusion, exorphins have repeatedly been shown to cause increased insulin production and release. Insulin is a hormone that moves glucose into cells. This means that many of the calories that celiacs absorb are likely to be stored as fat, rather than circulating in the blood and being available for energy demands. It is therefore not surprising that obesity has been found to be more common than wasting, among untreated celiac patients. Neither is it surprising that most untreated celiacs fall within the normal range for body mass, despite suffering from a disease involving malabsorption. The most sinister part of the increased insulin blood levels is that cancer cells need glucose for tumors to grow. This may explain the higher incidence of cancer reported in adult-onset, non-insulin dependent diabetes. The increased insulin production caused by gluten-derived exorphins not only masks malabsorption but also helps to feed tumors, accelerating their growth. The impact of exorphins on insulin production is likely another factor in the increased cancer rates among untreated celiacs.

THE ROOT OF THE CONFUSION

This confusing array of nutritional factors, and the signs that point to them, has some serious implications for diagnosing celiac patients. They also have some serious implications for many cancer patients. For instance, investigation of cancer patients for gluten sensitivity might offer new cause for hope. The evidence certainly suggests that a gluten-free diet can be very helpful to many cancer patients, but without suspecting and testing for gluten sensitivity, we will never know how many cancer-prone individuals the diet might help.

In summary, gluten consumption, in isolated groups, has been shown to increase the risk of cancer. Grain farming has also been shown to increase the risk of some cancers among grain farmers. Similarly, a gluten-free diet has been shown to reduce the risk of cancer in some of these groups. A gluten-free diet, sometimes in addition to elimination of other foods, has also been shown to be beneficial to cancer patients, especially in conjunction with conventional therapies. For many reasons—from morphine-like substances hidden in the proteins of these foods, to the nutrient deficiencies and abnormal intestinal permeability they cause, to the impact of exorphins on insulin production—gluten is a food that cancer patients should be urged to exclude from their diets.

Gluten consumption increased in the United States and Canada throughout the last century. Our increased consumption of processed foods and the diet fads touting high grains/carbohydrates has combined to encourage this steady increase. In parallel with the increased consumption of gluten grains, the rate of cancer deaths has risen from 2.5 percent in 1900 to nearly 30 percent, where it now rivals and will soon surpass cardiovascular disease as the primary cause of death in the United States. Given the evidence, a causative relationship between increased gluten consumption and cancer should be highly suspect.

The next several chapters combine to suggest why and how gluten cereals have managed to turn our immune systems against our own bodies—the system that is our primary defense mechanism against all disease.

Gluten, Molecular Mimicry, and Autoimmune Disease

Sixty-five to 68 percent of celiac children and adults have circulating antibodies that attack some of their own tissues—a characteristic of autoimmune disease. However, only 6 percent of normal subjects were found to have such autoantibodies. One group of researchers further reported that more than 20 percent of celiac patients had evidence of autoimmunity, including antithyroid and antipancreatic antibodies. A large majority of the celiac patients with these anti-self antibodies were not following a gluten-free diet. One of the most startling lessons we learned from our study of gluten sensitivity was that simply eliminating gluten from one's diet can reduce the body's production of these antibodies.

Further, given the elevated gliadin antibodies among patients with autoimmune diseases, in the absence of celiac disease, the evidence suggests that gluten sensitivity may be the most important factor that predisposes to autoimmune diseases. There are many autoimmune diseases that are affected by gluten, but we have chosen to explore just a few examples to demonstrate gluten's effect on the many forms of autoimmunity. We first show the overlap between autoimmunity and celiac disease, then a similar overlap with non-celiac gluten sensitivity. Finally, we report on the impact that a gluten-free diet has on the patients with specific autoimmune diseases and celiac disease. A gluten-free diet is often just as helpful to those non-celiacs who show only anti-gliadin antibodies and suffer from the same autoimmune disease.

Autoimmune diseases where gluten sensitivity and celiac disease should be ruled out include:

- Alopecia Areata (sudden head baldness confined to limited areas or patches)
- Arthritis
- Autoimmune thyroid disease
- Biliary atresia
- Biliary sclerosis
- Cirrhosis (of the liver)
- Crohn's disease
- Diabetes mellitus
- Fibromyalgia
- Hypoparathyroidism
- Idiopathic thrombocytopenic
- Microscopic colitis
- Multiple sclerosis
- Nephropathy (kidney disease)
- Optic neuritis
- Oral cankers (aphthous ulcers)
- purpura
- Sarcoidosis
- Systemic lupus erythematosus
- Trigeminal neuritis
- Vasculitis

CONNECTING AUTOIMMUNITY TO GLUTEN

The connection between autoimmune disease and gluten grains is supported by evidence that is clear and compelling. We have already established that gluten leaked into the bloodstream will injure a wide variety of human tissues. Such damage is likely a factor that leads to autoimmune disease, but that is far from the whole story. The risk of the many autoimmune disorders common in celiac disease increases with the length of time in which a celiac consumes gluten. Gluten sensitivity is also very common in patients with a variety of autoimmune diseases. Taken together, the evidence leaves little doubt that gluten is at least a factor in many, perhaps most cases of autoimmune diseases.

MOLECULAR MIMICRY

The most reasonable explanation we have found for the connection between gluten and autoimmune disease lies in a dynamic called "molecular mimicry," especially as it applies to food allergy. Molecular mimicry is driven by the fact that very different proteins are frequently made up of similar structures. When proteins that make up our own tissues appear similar to "invader" proteins, our immune systems will attack our own tissues. When foreign proteins, or large fragments of protein, enter the bloodstream, their presence is sensed by the immune system, which interprets them as non-self and potentially harmful. The immune system then begins production of antibodies that are specifically tailored to identify and destroy these invaders. These antibodies react just as they would to the foreign proteins of infectious agents such as bacteria and viruses. At the same time, the immune system also produces memory cells, which remember and recognize certain parts of the structure of this invader protein, should it enter the blood again.

The specific part of the protein sensed by the antibody is a set of amino acids. It is this set of amino acids, called an "epitope," to which the antibody attaches itself. Like a combination lock, these groups have a number of amino acids arranged in a specific order. The memory cells recognize the invader by the combination of amino acids in their protein structure and signal for rapid production of many antibodies. They are called antigen-specific antibodies because the immune system has constructed them to identify and attack only molecules with the identifying sequence. This process is the basis of vaccination and acquired immunity.

FOODS AND ABNORMAL ANTIBODY PRODUCTION

When we eat a food such as gluten (most Westerners eat it several times every day), we are likely to leak at least some incompletely digested, overly large proteins into our bloodstream, even when we are in good health. People prone to food allergy and gluten sensitivity are inclined to experience suppression of their digestive process, excessive leakiness of their gut lining, and an abnormal influx of partly digested foods. Even if the proteins are partly digested (due to the nature of the sulfide bonds holding gluten together, it is always poorly digested), the larger peptides from gluten are likely to contain a sequence that will result in production of specific memory cells.

If the small intestinal leakage continues on a day-to-day basis, antibody production will be kept at a very high level. This means that where there is daily gluten consumption, suppression of digestion, and a leaky gut, there will be excessive quantities of antibodies circulating throughout the body.

THE PROBLEM WITH CIRCULATING GLUTEN ANTIBODIES

Molecular mimicry, also called cross-reactivity, is thought to result in the formation of specific antibodies formed to protect us from our external environment—attacking internal molecules that display identical or very similar amino acid sequences. If these sequences in food molecules are duplicated in the structures that make up our own tissues, our antibodies will attack these look-alikes: Our immune system turns against us. Autoimmune diseases such as insulin-dependent diabetes mellitus (IDDM), thyroiditis, multiple sclerosis, and arthritis may be the end result. Alarmingly close similarities between gluten protein structure and the structure of body tissues have been reported, sometimes in association with particular autoimmune diseases. We can only conclude that chronic leakage of gluten proteins into the blood is a likely cause of autoimmune diseases.

GERMS AND MOLECULAR MIMICRY

Bacteria, viruses, and yeast probably do cause or contribute to at least some cases of autoimmune disease, but the evidence suggests that the majority of cases are, partly or wholly, the result of dietary proteins. Molecular mimicry requires chronic antibody production. So the trigger that starts and continues to signal the immune system to produce antibodies must be present on an ongoing basis. With a few exceptions, infectious agents that penetrate the body's defenses are either neutralized or destroyed by the immune system in a relatively short time. Dietary proteins such as gluten, on the other hand, are chronically present in the body, day after day. If the immune system reacts by making antibodies against this common food, then a gluten-containing diet may provide the necessary trigger to start an autoimmune disease, and to keep it going.

Conditions Necessary to Activate
Gluten-Induced Molecular Mimicry

1. regular consumption of gluten
2. a genetic predisposition, food allergy, or infectious assault that causes an abnormally permeable intestine or "leaky gut"
3. chronic absorption of large, incompletely digested molecules into the blood, whether proteins or partial proteins
4. antibody production that recognizes parts of dietary "non-self" protein structures

continued

---

5. identical or similar protein structures found naturally in our own self tissues
6. antibody attack of both self and non-self sequences

AUTOIMMUNE DISEASE AND GLUTEN SENSITIVITY

There are many autoimmune diseases where elevated antibodies against gluten are the rule rather than the exception. This can be interpreted as indicating that people with autoimmune disease have a more permeable intestine and that gluten is leaking into the blood and causing their autoimmunity through molecular mimicry. Or, it can be interpreted as indicating that gluten is causing an increase in their intestinal permeability and that other substances are being absorbed into the blood, causing their autoimmune disease. Either way, the presence of antibodies against gluten indicates that it is at least an important indicator of disease. The most reasonable response for anyone with an autoimmune disease and antibodies against gluten is the strict elimination of dietary gluten.

Now, let's have a careful look at four specific autoimmune diseases: autoimmune thyroid disease, insulin-dependent diabetes mellitus (IDDM), autoimmune liver disease, and rheumatoid arthritis, all of which occur more frequently in people with celiac disease and gluten sensitivity than in the general population (see appendix C for an extensive list of autoimmune diseases that occur more frequently with celiac disease and non-celiac gluten sensitivity).

AUTOIMMUNE THYROID DISEASE AND GLUTEN

Autoimmune thyroid disease can result in either overproduction or underproduction of thyroid hormones. Excessive thyroid production is found in almost 4.2 percent of people with celiac disease, and autoimmune underactivity of the thyroid gland is found in about 13 percent of celiac patients. This pattern is further supported by the data showing that other forms of thyroid disease that are not autoimmune are not significantly greater among celiacs. As with other autoimmune diseases, an increasing number of researchers are now recommending that all autoimmune thyroid patients be routinely screened for celiac disease.

From a different perspective, up to 4.8 percent of persons with autoimmune thyroid disease were found to have celiac disease. This is more than four times more common than the rate of celiac disease in nonautoimmune thyroid disease.

Whether celiac patients are tested for autoimmune thyroid disease, or people with autoimmune thyroid disease are tested for celiac disease, the result is that many more occurrences are found than in the general population. The overlap of these diseases speaks to the importance of recognizing that celiac disease and/or gluten sensitivity predispose people to autoimmune disease. Clearly, we need to be vigilant for such autoimmune diseases in newly diagnosed celiac patients. We also need to be vigilant for gluten sensitivity and celiac disease among those with autoimmune disease. A similar but more dramatic overlap is found in insulin-dependent diabetes.

INSULIN-DEPENDENT DIABETES MELLITUS (IDDM) AND GLUTEN

> **PLEASE NOTE:** After the complete autoimmune destruction of insulin-producing islet cells, a gluten-free diet does not reverse or stabilize IDDM. Gluten-induced neurological damage is also commonly irreversible.

While less than ½ of 1 percent of all Americans have insulin-dependent diabetes mellitus (IDDM), as many as 10 percent of all celiacs develop IDDM, and up to 8 percent of IDDM patients have or will develop celiac disease. Many authorities are now emphatically recommending that all IDDM patients be screened annually for celiac disease after the initial IDDM diagnosis. There are 1 million IDDM patients in the United States today, with approximately thirty thousand patients diagnosed each year.

Clearly, there is considerable overlap between celiac disease and IDDM. It is well established that celiac disease is the direct result of gluten. Our first clue that gluten may be a major cause of diabetes is found in the overlap of the occurrence of celiac disease and IDDM.

A recent report indicates that IDDM is generally on the rise, especially in populations that previously enjoyed low rates of this disease. We suspect that this reflects worldwide increases in consumption of the diabetogenic foods—gluten, soy, and cow's milk. Further, Finland and Sardinia are reporting two of the highest rates of IDDM in the world. These are two of the three areas with the highest rates of celiac disease.

GROUP	PREVALENCE OF CELIAC DISEASE
Saharawi Muslim adolescents in Morocco	1 in 18
Northern Sardinia	1 in 70
Finland	1 in 85

From animal studies, we now know that among rats that are genetically susceptible to IDDM, feeding wheat gluten will cause 40 percent to develop IDDM. Several other groups of rats with the same genetic inclination to develop IDDM were fed gluten-free diets, and only 10 to 15 percent of these groups developed IDDM. Further, the rate and severity of diabetes could be manipulated by varying the amount of gluten in the diet. Others have shown that delaying introduction of dietary gluten in animal models delays or prevents diabetes. Most authorities in this area of diabetes research conclude that gluten is a major factor in causing the development of IDDM in genetically predisposed animals.

This work, along with other research over the past decade, has some serious implications for an emerging therapy for IDDM patients. For example, a series of medical advances have made it possible to transplant insulin-producing cells into diabetic patients. There are three major difficulties in this dramatic medical advance. First, when full insulin production is achieved, it is only temporary and lasts for an unpredictable period of time. The second problem is that these transplants usually result in only partial insulin production. A third concern is that the same autoimmune insulin-producing cellular destruction may occur if these transplanted diabetic patients continue to eat a gluten- or soy-rich diabetogenic diet. We believe that the patients receiving these islet cell transplants would benefit from excluding gluten, soy, and dairy products from their diet.

Multiple Sclerosis–Diabetes Connection

Some startling new research has revealed that the overlap between multiple sclerosis (MS) and IDDM is so great that they may simply be different manifestations of the same disease. We have long understood that MS patients produce antibodies that attack their own myelin, the insulating sheath on nerve fibers. MS researchers are now reporting that many MS antibodies will attack insulin-producing cells. Further, they also report that antibodies from most IDDM patients will attack the myelin sheath on nerves. We anxiously await confirmation of these results and suspect that it is yet another point of convergence between gluten and these two autoimmune diseases.

Type 2, Non-Insulin-Dependent Diabetes

The current explosion of Type 2 diabetes among our young people points to an indirect result of our culture's gluten gluttony. Loading the diet with so much carbohydrate (dominated by cereal grains) leads to down-regulation of cellular insulin receptors. This chronic carbohydrate consumption and, hence, elevated blood sugar, have to cause excessive insulin production, along with a tendency to overproduce the pro-inflammatory, pro-cancer, pro-allergy, pro-cardiovascular disease, metabolism inhibiting prostaglandin E2 series.

Both celiac disease and diabetes are major contributors to the epidemic of magnesium deficiency and chromium deficiency. Up to 90 percent of Americans and Canadians consume less than the minimal 50 micrograms of chromium a day. It follows that celiacs eating a normal diet would be profoundly chromium deficient. Chromium deficiency is associated with

1. hyperglycemia
2. hyperinsulinism/insulin-resistance
3. insulin-dependent diabetes (IDDM, Type 1)
4. adult-onset diabetes (NIDDM, Type 2)
5. gestational diabetes (diabetes of pregnancy)
6. corticosteroid-induced diabetes
7. excessive body fat/lowered lean body weight
8. elevated total cholesterol
9. elevated LDL cholesterol
10. elevated apolipoprotein B
11. lowered HDL cholesterol
12. lowered apolipoprotein A-1
13. atherosclerosis
14. syndrome X (central [abdominal] obesity, diabetes, elevated cholesterol, high blood pressure, elevated triglycerides, etc.)

15. alcohol abuse
16. excessive consumption of refined sugars and cereals

AUTOIMMUNE LIVER DISEASE AND GLUTEN

Chronic liver disease of unknown cause is common in celiac patients, and a gluten-free diet usually results in improvements in liver enzyme profiles along with resolution of the liver disease. Some researchers recommend testing for celiac disease in cases where there is no known reason for elevated liver enzymes, reporting that 9 percent of these patients have celiac disease. Other reports indicate high levels of gliadin antibodies among patients with liver disease in the absence of celiac disease.

Many individuals suffering from a range of liver diseases, including biliary cirrhosis and chronic active hepatitis, have elevated anti-gliadin antibodies in their blood. As many as 11 to 20 percent of patients with cirrhosis and chronic hepatitis, depending on the type of liver disease, are gluten sensitive. Yet, it was only among the patients with autoimmune hepatitis that there was an increase in celiac disease.

Because cases of liver disease occurring in conjunction with celiac disease usually show dramatic improvement or complete remission on a gluten-free diet, the connection with gluten is difficult to deny. It also suggests the potential value of excluding gluten even among those who are non-celiac gluten sensitive. The common misguided assumption that elevated gliadin antibodies are meaningless or coincidental without biopsy-proven celiac disease is inappropriate, and we think this assumption is harmful to the patient. Dismissal of such results denies the patient the opportunity to benefit from further testing or a gluten-free diet.

RHEUMATOID ARTHRITIS AND GLUTEN

Rheumatoid Arthritis Alleviated by a Gluten-Free Diet

started developing rheumatoid arthritis in 1990. By 1994 I could hardly walk in the mornings. My hip joints were extremely stiff. I could only shuffle forward and could not pivot my right hip.

My family doctor said that I would need a hip replacement operation someday. It was then that I started doing research into gluten sensitivity, really on behalf of my mother, who suffers from Crohn's disease. When I was reading about Crohn's disease, I discovered that not only Crohn's but also many other ailments were being researched in the United Kingdom and United States in relation to gluten. The more I read, the more I realized that all these symptoms were in my family.

I visited a registered dietitian and posed the questions: "Could I be 'allergic' to gluten? Will I get Crohn's disease like my mother?" The dietitian suggested that I go on a gluten-free diet for two weeks, then test myself with a lot of gluten over three or four days. What I discovered then has changed my life forever! My sinusitis was completely gone in five to six months. My chronic constipation, which I had suffered since childhood, went away. I now take no medication whatsoever. When I realized that I had saved myself a hip replacement operation, I decided to start a support group. I decided that there were many people that a change in eating habits would help. I now work very hard to bring this information to as many people as I can. It really is a message that needs to be taken to everyone.

Lucille C.

The studies in medical literature on rheumatoid arthritis (RA) and juvenile chronic arthritis reveal both a relationship between these diseases and gluten and some shocking facts about how often celiac disease and gluten sensitivity are likely to be overlooked in many cases of these joint diseases. This literature is also somewhat of an exposé of the devastating potential of gluten grains. Children with hauntingly painful and horribly disfigured joints often wait years to be tested for celiac disease. When they finally are tested, they will often test positive. For them, relief follows the gluten-free diet, although their disfigured joints will likely serve as permanent reminders of that pain.

Researchers are reporting the occurrence of celiac disease over five times more frequently among people with rheumatoid arthritis. The prevalence ranged as high as 7.5 percent. That is an occurrence that should grab anyone's attention. More remarkably, about half of the patients with rheumatoid arthritis show clear signs of gluten sensitivity through elevated serum levels of anti-gliadin antibodies. More specifically, a variety of antibody blood tests has revealed non-celiac gluten sensitivity in 34 percent of juvenile chronic arthritis patients and in 47 percent of adult rheumatoid arthritics.

Although such elevated antibody levels were long considered to be the result of increased intestinal permeability caused by non-steroidal anti-inflammatory drug (NSAID) pain management, there is now solid evidence to counter this view. One study compared anti-gliadin antibody levels from RA patients early in their disease with those who have advanced disease. They found that anti-gliadin antibodies are elevated in 48 percent of the patients who have recently developed arthritis, while only 25 percent of those with advanced disease show elevated gliadin antibodies. They suggest that their results may point to a gluten factor that begins this destructive inflammatory joint disease in these patients. We agree.

Reports of arthritis, after the discovery of celiac disease, indicate that the arthritis pain either improves or completely resolves on a gluten-free diet. There is often little need for pain relief after a few months on the diet. There are only a very few exceptions where the condition continues to progress, perhaps due to some mechanism that becomes independent of gluten, making the condition chronic. One group investigated the impact of fasting followed by a gluten-free, vegetarian diet (not what we would recommend) on a group of rheumatoid arthritis patients. They reported significant objective and subjective benefits.

The agonies imposed by arthritis require medications for pain management that risk significant, often debilitating, side effects, including kidney failure, bleeding ulcers, perforation of the intestine, acceleration of joint destruction after ten years on medication, and early death. Yet many arthritis patients are reported to suffer for two to fifteen years before they are finally tested for celiac disease. A cursory viewing of the X rays of these patients' joints is heart wrenching, and such delays seem needlessly cruel.

It is difficult to imagine a rational argument against first ruling out celiac disease and non-celiac gluten sensitivity, especially when they are both found so frequently in many types of arthritis. Yet, individuals with gluten-caused or aggravated rheumatoid arthritis may never be told— may never be given the option of the diet because non-celiac gluten sensitivity is too often dismissed as "nonspecific."

We strongly urge the routine blood testing of all arthritis patients for delayed-onset food allergy and gluten sensitivity, and, if allergic foods are identified, strict exclusion of those foods should be prescribed.

Both Food and Infection May Contribute to Rheumatoid Arthritis

To further complicate the issue, one group of researchers has presented evidence revealing that a combination of dietary protein and bacteria contributes to the progression of rheumatoid arthritis. Diet-induced intestinal permeability allows leakage of "friendly" bacteria from the intestine into the bloodstream, where it travels to, and becomes bound to, joint tissues. The immune system attacks, damaging both the intestinal bacteria and the joint tissues to which these bacteria are bound.

CANCER CONVERGENCE WITH OTHER AILMENTS IN CELIAC DISEASE

People with autoimmune disease have increased risk of celiac disease, as do intravenous drug users. Celiac patients also experience an increased risk of cancer and autoimmune diseases. While these occurrences may seem unrelated, these associations actually point to an important issue when looking at cancer risk.

In autoimmunity and celiac disease there is increased intestinal permeability, allowing leakage of partly digested proteins into the blood, many of which have repeatedly been shown to have opioid activity. Many addicts, of course, inject opiates directly into the bloodstream or tissues adjacent to blood vessels. These food-derived peptides and infected drugs have an important feature in common: They signal natural killer cells in our immune system to slow or stop their normal activities. Through this process, called "downregulation," we lose the activity of the very cells that are the body's first line of defense against disease and, in particular, malignancy. Due to this opioid activity, our immune system is inhibited from identifying and destroying the body's tissue cells that have damaged or fragile chromosomes, thus preventing them from becoming cancerous.

MODEL FOR THE DIETARY TREATMENT OF AUTOIMMUNITY

The evidence presented here indicates that routine testing for celiac disease and gluten sensitivity should be conducted on all patients with autoimmune disease. The evidence also suggests that treatment with a gluten-free diet may offer dramatic improvements far beyond those offered by medications aimed at pain control or down-regulating the immune system. Dietary therapies, although more controversial, do not cause the often unpleasant, and sometimes very dangerous, side effects associated with drugs, especially those used for pain management.

A study on psoriasis (a very unpleasant autoimmune skin disease) serves as a model for connecting gluten with autoimmunity. Several anecdotal reports suggested that psoriasis might be more frequent in celiac disease. But, when investigated, the connection was not supported. Testing of a group of 302 patients with psoriasis revealed that 16 percent showed at least one type of antibody against gliadin. Within this group, two patients had celiac disease, or approaching 1 percent, which is reflective of the general population. However, these researchers then enrolled the non-celiac gluten-sensitive patients with psoriasis in a dietary study. Of the thirty patients who stayed with the strict gluten-free diet, the entire group showed a significant decrease in the signs and symptoms of psoriasis. When they returned to a regular diet, as part of the study, more than half of these people experienced a resurgence of psoriatic symptoms. The report unequivocally recommends a gluten-free diet as a treatment for psoriasis patients who have anti-gliadin antibodies.

CONCLUSION

Celiac disease and non-celiac gluten sensitivity often underlie autoimmune disease. Gluten is the common thread that connects many forms of autoimmunity, including the four types of autoimmunity that we have used as examples to demonstrate this connection.

A majority of those with untreated celiac disease show at least some indication of additional forms of autoimmunity. Further, autoimmune thyroid disease is overrepresented among those with celiac disease, and celiac disease is overrepresented among those who have any form of autoimmune thyroid disease. A similar overlap is seen in insulin-dependent diabetes mellitus, autoimmune liver disease, and rheumatoid arthritis.

Of at least equal importance is that non-celiac gluten sensitivity is also overrepresented among those with these autoimmune diseases. Although the connections between celiac disease and autoimmunity are well documented, the celiac patient must often be proactive and request appropriate testing and follow-up.

Unfortunately, celiac disease and non-celiac gluten sensitivity are often differentiated, which may lead to less satisfactory medical advice. Positive test results showing gluten sensitivity may be dismissed on the assumption that such results are nonspecific. Patients may not be encouraged to follow a strict gluten-free diet. More commonly, their immune reactions to gluten may never even be mentioned.

In autoimmune disease, we recommend testing for both celiac disease and gluten sensitivity. When patients have positive antibody tests for either, a gluten-free diet should be followed.

Osteoporosis and Gluten

I was diagnosed about thirteen years ago with celiac. I weighed 112 pounds, and I am six feet one inch tall. I was still walking/ working, but barely. I had stress fractures in my feet. My vision had deteriorated to the point where I was getting a new prescription about every six months. I was having nosebleeds every day along with headaches, abdominal cramps, leg cramps, muscle twitching, tingling in my fingers and toes, bone pain, etc. About three days after going gluten free, I felt better. I had to get new prescriptions on my glasses about every six months due to vision improvement. My hair grew back. I gained about 60 pounds over three years.

Jim B.

If you have weak, porous bones, you might want to eliminate gluten from your diet even if you do not mount an immune response to this food. A significant portion of our society is plagued by this silent disability. The first painful hint of a problem is often a broken bone. There are several ways that gluten can interfere with maintaining strong, healthy bones. In this chapter, we explain how gluten can cause this crippling and painful malady.

According to the National Osteoporosis Foundation, osteoporosis is a major public health threat for more than 28 million Americans, 80 percent of whom are women. In the United States today, 8 million women and 2 million men already have osteoporosis, and 18 million more have low bone density, placing them at increased risk for osteoporosis; hip, back, and wrist fractures; and premature death.

Approximately 250,000 Americans die annually from the complications associated with hip fractures. Co-author James Braly's father was one such osteoporotic hip fracture victim.

Cases of bone degeneration are increasing at an epidemic rate. Much of it is due to our aging population, of course, with women now living well beyond eighty and men following closely behind. But that is only part of the explanation. Current dietary recommendations are shortsighted and out of date, reflecting a simplistic view of the many factors that contribute to building and maintaining strong, healthy bones.

The source of much of this poor advice is the infamous USDA food guide pyramid. Its proponents have failed to keep pace with current research. Despite exploding numbers of cases of osteoporosis and the well-documented, negative impact of gluten consumption on bone density, daily consumption of six to eleven servings of cereal is still recommended. Such recommendations are akin to urging a drowning man to drink more water. These recommendations are a clear denial of much of what we now know about bones, how they grow, and what makes them strong.

GLUTEN CAN ALSO CAUSE OSTEOPOROSIS IN THE NON-GLUTEN SENSITIVE

Phytate is the storage form of most phosphorus found in plants. It has a strong attraction to a variety of minerals including calcium, magnesium, iron, and zinc. Even for people who do not suffer from gluten sensitivity, phytates are cause for concern. They are found in large quantities in the outer layer of cereal grains. During digestion, especially in the stomach, phytates will combine with calcium and other minerals. The bonds that form in these chemical combinations are resistant to the human digestive process, so important minerals will be wasted when phytates are consumed. Therefore, by eating whole grains we decrease the availability of those dietary minerals that help us grow and maintain strong, healthy bones.

GLUTEN, VITAMINS, AND BONE HEALTH

Further, grain consumption often displaces fruits and vegetables that are good sources of some important vitamins needed to keep our bones healthy. Vitamin C contributes to bone maintenance by aiding in the production of collagen. Production of this connective tissue is needed not only for the repair of bone breaks but also for the replacement of aging collagen that is destroyed by osteoclasts in the normal turnover of bone tissues.

Vitamin K is deficient in the diets of many women, many celiacs, and most people suffering from osteoporosis. At one time, vitamin K, an essential vitamin derived from food and the action of intestinal bacteria, was thought to be involved solely with the clotting of blood. As it turns out, vitamin K is needed in other key processes, including the production of osteocalcin by osteoblasts. Osteocalcin is a bone protein important in bone metabolism and bone formation. When excessive levels are found in the blood, it is associated with bone disorders such as Paget's disease and postmenopausal osteoporosis.

The January 1999 issue of the *American Journal of Clinical Nutrition* reported on more than seventy-two thousand women who were divided on the basis of their consumption of vitamin K. Those who consumed the most vitamin K were only 70 percent as likely to have broken a hip as women in the group that took in the least amount of this important vitamin. More impressive was the observation of lettuce consumption. Women who ate vitamin K–rich lettuce at least once a day were 45 percent less likely to have a hip fracture than those who ate the same food once a week or less. Consuming less than 109 micrograms of vitamin K resulted in bone thinning, but more than 109 micrograms did not add any more protection against hip fracture.

For women ages fifteen and older, federal guidelines recommend consuming 180 micrograms of vitamin K each day, probably an excessive amount. On the other hand, the RDA for vitamin K is 65 micrograms for women and 80 micrograms for men, which is probably too low.

The research findings clearly demonstrate that other nutrients besides calcium are important for maintaining healthy bones. Instead of the current narrow focus on calcium, women ought to be sure to eat a well-balanced diet containing enough protein and vitamin K. In addition to broccoli, lettuce, and other leafy vegetables, foods rich in vitamin K include pork, liver, and vegetable oils.

Vitamin A deficiency, another problem that often arises from gluten consumption, can cause stunted growth in children and can also impact on adult bones. Because this vitamin coordinates both bone-building and bone-destroying cells, a deficiency may cause a wide range of bone abnormalities. To ensure sufficient vitamin A in your diet, eat foods such as fish, flax, and liver, which are rich in this important vitamin.

BONES ARE VERY MUCH ALIVE

Bones are living tissue. Calcium, magnesium, zinc, and other minerals are deposited and removed on an ongoing basis. Connective tissues within bones and supporting the bones are renewed regularly. This work is conducted by cells that are bone builders (osteoblasts) and cells that are bone destroyers (osteoclasts). Our bones are made up of about 25 percent water, 25 percent protein, and the rest are mineral salts, mostly calcium. Collagen is the connective tissue that provides the flexible framework on which these brittle mineral salts crystallize. In healthy bones, this combination results in strong, somewhat flexible bones. The minerals provide rigidity, and the collagen provides flexibility while reinforcing the minerals, much like the principles that give reinforced concrete its strength.

WHAT IS OSTEOPOROSIS?

When our bones are broken by mild impact or by normal, day-to-day stresses, they are not healthy. Weak bones usually have more and larger spaces between the mineral crystals that weaken bones by making them porous. By now, it will be no surprise for you to learn that gluten can cause this terrible, debilitating condition. Contrary to the current, unfortunate dietary fad, dairy products may also be contributing to many cases of osteoporosis.

Adult-diagnosed celiacs invariably suffer some degree of demineralization of their bones. The extent of this damage can be quite dramatic.

WHAT CAUSES OSTEOPOROSIS IN CELIAC PATIENTS?

For a long time, it was assumed that widespread osteoporosis among celiacs was the result of malabsorption. While it makes sense that we would be unable to absorb enough calcium, resulting in a deficiency, when researchers looked more closely at this issue they found that the evidence doesn't support such a simplistic view. It seems that gluten has a greater impact on calcium metabolism than on actual absorption because it increases how much calcium we waste after it is absorbed. A gluten-free diet often results in dramatic improvements to the mineral content of celiac patients' bones, but this is largely due to increased retention of calcium.

A related paradox of osteoporosis and celiac disease is that calcium supplementation does not help to remineralize celiac patients' bones as much as magnesium supplementation. There is comparatively much less magnesium in our bones, so this information provides an important clue to the fascinating puzzle of the impact that gluten can have on bone density.

Not only is magnesium important to the activation of bone-building osteoblasts that deposit calcium and add collagen to our bones but is also a factor that aids in repairing the parathyroid gland. This is a gland that produces the hormones (PTH) that regulate most of the body's calcium metabolism. These hormones signal the kidneys to recover calcium from the urine, to elevate blood levels of calcium, and to activate vitamin D (calcitrol), which signals the intestine to absorb calcium from the food we eat. Clearly, adequate dietary calcium is of little value if we are not getting enough magnesium for the parathyroid gland to function properly.

For these reasons, dairy products and calcium supplementation may actually have a negative impact on the density of our bones, exactly the opposite of what we were taught to expect. It also counters the simplistic advice to consume calcium supplements alone and/or dairy products that are often offered to many individuals with declining bone density. Magnesium, calcium, zinc, boron, and vitamins D and K, all reported to be deficient in many celiacs, are absorbed from the intestine by the same mechanism, called "active transport." Loading the digestive tract with calcium alone overwhelming invites this part of our absorptive capacity with a single mineral, albeit the most common one in the body. This approach is shortsighted and, quite frankly, harmful. It risks causing a deficiency of magnesium and other necessary minerals, which are less abundant and frequently deficient in our diets. Magnesium and phosphorous deficiencies caused by excessive calcium intake may pose a much greater risk of causing bone mineral loss. Further, the risk is largely independent of the traditional suspect in gluten-induced bone damage—

malabsorption. The key issue is the balance of relative quantities in which these minerals are available, either in our diets and/or the supplements we consume.

Great care should be taken in recommending calcium supplementation, especially among those who already suffer from bone demineralization and among those at greatest risk of developing such problems. A typical, healthy intestine only absorbs a small portion of the calcium that is available from our food. At the same time, evidence suggests that excess calcium intake competes with magnesium absorption, further aggravating a poor magnesium status. Flooding our diet with more and more calcium is a dangerously simplistic approach to this complex problem.

Many hospital emergency rooms are now using large therapeutic doses of intravenous magnesium as one of the first-line therapies for cardiac patients. Such magnesium treatments have been shown to reduce the extent of damage to the heart muscles and tissues. More and more medical clinics and emergency rooms are also beginning to use IV magnesium as a first-line therapy to abort migraine headaches and asthma attacks. The effectiveness of these therapies also suggests a common condition of chronic magnesium deficiency. We view this common deficiency as a predictable result of our culture's obsession with magnesium-depleting consumption of massive quantities of dairy products and cereal grains.

THE PARATHYROID GLAND

Recall that, in untreated celiac disease, the parathyroid gland releases an excess of parathyroid hormone, the single most important hormone for regulating calcium metabolism. This is associated with abnormally high bone turnover and bone loss. We now have evidence that, at least in some cases of celiac disease, endomysium antibodies (the same ones that are sought in screening tests for celiac disease) will cross-react with parathyroid tissues, resulting in damage to this important gland and compromising its ability to effectively regulate our calcium metabolism. Thinning of the bone, increased bone fragility, and proneness to low-impact bone fractures are the consequences.

The tragic underdiagnosis of celiac disease and gluten sensitivity certainly suggests the need for more frequent screening for these conditions among those with reduced bone density. Such testing should be conducted as early as possible to allow early and extensive gains in mineral deposition, resulting in strong, healthy bones prior to declining production of sex hormones and growth hormones later in life.

OSTEOMALACIA AND GLUTEN

Another bone-density ailment that can also be related to gluten consumption is osteomalacia. This is a condition where the bones are very flexible and weak. There appears to be ample collagen, but calcium, phosphorus, and/or other necessary minerals for bone hardness are lacking. The childhood equivalent of osteomalacia is rickets. Both are often the result of deficiencies in vitamin D. Recall that it is the active form of vitamin D, calcitrol, that signals the intestine to absorb more calcium and other minerals from our food.

In osteomalacia and its milder form, osteopenia, our bones bend and become deformed due to a deficiency of absorbed minerals, and this condition can often be halted and reversed by simple vitamin D supplementation. Unfortunately, bone deformations usually are not corrected. Those who get little exposure to unimpeded sunlight, perhaps due to their jobs, age, or medical condition, are at risk. Those who live in temperate zones of the world run a seasonal risk of developing this problem.

Impaired kidney function, where there is excessive calcium excretion, can also result in rickets, osteomalacia, and osteopenia. There is clear evidence that gluten contributes to at least some cases of impaired kidney function.

THE IMPACT OF AGING AND SEX HORMONES ON BONE HEALTH

All of the above factors in building and maintaining dense, healthy bones become increasingly important as we approach middle age. The sex hormones estrogen and testosterone stimulate the action of bone-building osteoblasts. As women experience menopause and men approach their sixties, production of these sex hormones is reduced. Bone building therefore slows and begins to be outstripped by bone destruction. If we have built up strong bones in our early years, if we continue with weight-bearing exercise regularly, and if we are eating and absorbing adequate quantities and an appropriate balance of all the necessary minerals, our bones should continue to serve us throughout our old age. If we are gluten sensitive or have celiac disease, even if religiously pursuing a gluten-free diet, we may need to take aggressive action, supplementing magnesium and ensuring adequate vitamin D intake or absorption.

If you have a personal history of osteoporosis or osteopenia, periodic bone-density tests should be done to assure that your gluten-free diet and supplementation program are working optimally for you.

BACK TO THE FUTURE

Gluten and dairy products are two of the most allergenic foods in our food supply. As we have shown, calcium supplements as a primary or sole nutrient intervention and consumption of gluten and dairy products can actually threaten our absorption of other important minerals, compromise our bones and general health, and cause the very disease they are purported to prevent.

As you have seen, there are many factors that affect bone health. Regular exercise, ample sunshine, a varied non-allergenic diet, and a variety of vitamins are needed, along with several important minerals and hormones. All of these factors must work in a balanced, harmonious manner to build and maintain strong bones. Any change in this balance can lead to sudden and measurable changes in a relatively short time. Substantial improvements in bone density occur within one year of diagnosing celiac disease and beginning a gluten-free diet. Excessive calcium supplementation, without a balance of other bone nutrients, may well contribute to the very problem that it is aimed at helping.

A gluten-free, dairy-free diet that includes a wide range of meats, organ meat, fish, poultry, vegetables, and fruits, with moderate quantities of non-gluten grains, is not only closer to the one we evolved to eat but also one that will give us strong, healthy bones. Given the importance of an optimally functioning parathyroid gland for bone health, the cross-reaction between endomysium antibodies and the parathyroid gland also suggests that there may be autoimmune factors contributing to the bone damage caused by gluten.

Brain Disorders
and Gluten

Modern gluten gluttony has even invaded the private recesses of our minds. In this chapter we outline many of the psychiatric and neurological problems that can result from gluten sensitivity. The elimination of dietary gluten might soon replace many more expensive and ponderously slow conventional psychiatric treatments.

A BRIEF HISTORY OF GLUTEN'S EFFECTS ON MENTAL HEALTH

As many celiacs will attest, periods of fasting will provide at least a partial recovery from the symptoms of celiac disease, including relieving chronic depression and sleeping problems, and cause a strong overall sense of psychological well-being. There are many cases throughout history demonstrating the impact of diet on mental health. Starvation was used in ancient Greece to treat insanity. More tellingly, during World War II, the prevalence of schizophrenia dropped precipitously among European populations where there were grain shortages. If schizophrenia is, in large part, the result of gluten-derived opioids, the ancient strategy of fasting might well be quite an effective short-term strategy.

A very active research group at the Royal Hallamshire Hospital in Sheffield, involving the departments of neurology, gastroenterology, and histopathology, has demonstrated that gluten is a factor in a wide range of neurological conditions. More than half of the fifty-three patients with neurological conditions of unknown causes showed antibodies against gliadin. Of these thirty patients, nine had celiac disease. The other twenty-one of these patients were obviously gluten sensitive.

THE WIDE RANGE OF THE NEUROLOGICAL EFFECTS OF GLUTEN

What must it be like to live your life never knowing if, just at a critical or dangerous moment, you will have a seizure? Imagine the sense of uncertainty and vulnerability. Or what must it be like to experience the daily corrosion of what was once a good memory? What must it feel like to lose the ability to walk? Or the ability to talk? Worse yet, what must it feel like to experience an internal world that is partly made of visual and auditory hallucinations but is also partly the external objective world that others share? These are only a few of the many powerfully negative neurological consequences of eating gluten.

Many common brain diseases are known to be associated with high rates of both celiac disease and non-celiac gluten sensitivity. These include ataxia, peripheral neuropathies, or other such "chronic neurological conditions of unknown cause" (note: most chronic neurological conditions are of unknown cause). This also includes senility, another extremely common brain disorder that often appears to be related to gluten sensitivity. In senility, however, one has to catch and treat the mental deterioration early in order to prevent its progression. Unfortunately, continued deterioration despite a gluten-free diet is common in late-stage senility. For this reason, we will focus on prevention, through early detection and treatment of gluten sensitivity.

While the disorders of degeneration, blood circulation, and seizures can alter behavior, emotions, and learning, there are many more conditions that are affected by gluten. Psychological depression, neurotransmitter deficiencies, autism, and hyperactivity disorders can also be brought on by gluten sensitivity. These other brain diseases are associated with important changes to the brain, but, unlike epilepsy and senility, there is no visible structural brain damage. The evidence points to the action of gluteomorphin, a morphinelike substance that is derived from dietary gluten, as an important cause of these conditions.

You may want to examine your genetic heritage and determine whether you might be at risk. But the first step is to understand how gluten and its derivatives affect the brain, then to have a careful look at the specific behavioral, psychiatric, and neurological conditions that have been connected to gluten.

ANTI-GLUTEN ANTIBODIES THAT ATTACK THE BRAIN

We know that hallucinations, epilepsy, and disordered blood supply within the brain are easily explained by the actions of gluten or its derivatives. There is mounting evidence that these abnormalities may be the result of the interaction between our immune systems, gluten, and self-tissues. In blood taken from untreated celiac patients, researchers found antibodies that attack blood vessel walls in the human brain. Only three individuals in the control group showed gluten sensitivity, but none of this latter group showed antibodies as did the above untreated celiac patients.

Relatedly, when cats are fed gluten, they develop structural abnormalities in the brain. Celiac patients experience a wide range of neurological ailments that have also been shown to involve changes to the brain's structure.

Taken together, this evidence suggests that the antibodies of celiac patients sometimes enter the brain, where they can cause irreversible damage in some cases of epilepsy, chronic schizophrenia, and progressive neurological conditions. In other cases, such as newly diagnosed or newly relapsed schizophrenia, epilepsy, and disordered blood distribution in the brain, there may be a rapid improvement on a gluten-free diet.

ERGOTISM

Even the molds that grow on gluten grains have proven to pose a serious neurological and mental-health threat. Ergot is a fungus that will grow on any of the gluten-containing grains when they become damp for an extended period, but it is most frequently found on rye. Ergot poisoning, or ergotism, was known in the late Middle Ages as St. Anthony's Fire. People suffering from St. Anthony's Fire were sometimes accused of witchcraft because of the seizures and hallucinations caused by ergot. This reaction to ergot is not surprising, considering that this mold is the source from which the hallucinogenic drug LSD is refined.

Although ergotism occasionally afflicts domestic livestock, resulting in neurological symptoms, and sometimes lameness and death, modern grain-processing techniques usually provide good protection against it. Grains used for human consumption are now treated with much more care. Today, people are rarely afflicted with ergotism, and then it is usually due to overuse of certain drugs intentionally derived from rye molds grown in the laboratory. Such drugs are sometimes used to treat the excessive expansion of blood vessels in the brain that usually underlies migraine headaches. In fact, rye-mold derived ergot is such an effective constrictor of blood vessels that ergotism often results in lameness, followed by gangrenous tissue decay due to the poor circulation to the affected limb.

Peptides derived from gluten grains have since been implicated in schizophrenia, epileptic seizures, and vascular illnesses and are sometimes found to occur among patients who also have celiac disease. Like ergot, these peptides have recently been shown to affect blood flow within the brain, attention deficit hyperactivity disorder, and autism. Taken together, this information clearly suggests the connection between bioactive peptides derived from grains and the many disorders that also manifest gluten antibodies.

MOOD, BEHAVIOR, PSYCHOLOGY, AND GLUTEN

When looking at the kinds of brain and neurological injuries and ailments commonly found in celiac disease and gluten-sensitive patients, one finds extremely interesting and important patterns. Mood is often reflected in behavior. Disturbances of mood have long been recognized in celiac patients. From the very earliest reports, statements such as the following have characterized celiac children:

> The temper of the child seems variable, most frequently he is extremely irritable, fretful, capricious, or peevish. Nothing seems to please him, and altogether he is quite unlike himself.

This is a sentiment that has been repeated frequently in literature and continues to be mentioned by researchers. One report indicates that 63 percent of celiac children present with aggressive, bullying, angry, or irritable behavior.

Depression has been claimed as the most common symptom of celiac disease. Some researchers argue for routine blood testing for celiac disease on the basis of behavioral disturbance or depression alone. Whether we look at depression, anxiety, or behavior problems, such psychiatric symptoms are often eliminated by the simple removal of gluten from the diet.

Even among those with silent or asymptomatic celiac disease, a gluten-free diet often improves psychological well-being. In fact, some researchers are recommending that celiac disease be recognized as a bio-psycho-social disorder. Other researchers have warned that symptoms that appear to be caused by psychological factors, such as recurring complaints of stomachaches and irritability after the birth of a younger sibling, may be the result of unrecognized celiac disease.

Attention Deficit Disorder
(with or without Hyperactivity)

Disorders of mood and mind are also common in people who experience difficulty in maintaining their attention, but the most prominent feature of attention deficit disorder is the inability to maintain focus and attention where there is not a strong emotional motive. Whether the afflicted individual is lethargically disinterested in her or his surroundings or is hyperactive and unable to settle into a task, the attention-challenged individual in question may well be suffering from gluten sensitivity.

About 70 percent of children with untreated celiac disease show exactly the same abnormalities in brain-wave patterns as those who have been diagnosed with attention deficit disorder. Another recent study, the first of its kind, reported that food allergens, including wheat, could reproducibly cause abnormal brain waves. The most remarkable part of this research is that it shows that after a year of excluding gluten from the diet, all of these abnormalities disappear. For these children, diet not only treats their celiac disease but also their brains and ADD.

Celiac children also show dramatic improvements in mood after a short time on the diet. Since celiac disease afflicts about 1 percent of the population, and gluten sensitivity afflicts many more people, and since there are identical abnormalities in the brain-wave patterns of celiac children and ADHD children, it seems likely that there is a significant overlap between these groups. Given the evidence for overlap with gluten sensitivity, we think it is very likely that many people afflicted with attention deficits would benefit from a gluten-free, food allergen–free diet.

Learning Problems and Gluten Sensitivity

The learning problems associated with celiac disease and immune re-actions to milk proteins are related but separate issues. One study looked for dyslexia, a learning disorder marked by an inability to recognize and comprehend written words, in 291 fourth-grade children. Of the fifteen children who were determined to have dyslexia, two were subsequently diagnosed with celiac disease, and one had antibodies against milk pro-tein. If these findings reflect the rates of celiac disease and/or milk protein intolerance among dyslexic children, then diet may offer a powerful rem-edy for dyslexia. These children were placed on a gluten- and dairy-free diet, but follow-up data are not yet available.

Other learning disabilities, including both short-term auditory memory and slow visual processing speed, are much more common in celiac disease than in the general population, especially among male patients. We can only speculate about what such a diet might offer to those dyslexics who do not show immune reactions to these foods, but the evidence appears to warrant blood tests and a personal experiment. Dyslexia is a condition that has lifelong career implications and can have a powerful impact on self-esteem.

Alcoholism and Gluten

Inspired by the work of Theron Randolph, M.D., Joan Matthews-Larson, author of *Seven Weeks to Sobriety*, has reported significant food aller-gies in 73 of the 100 alcoholics she studied. She also reported that Herbert Karolus, M.D., found that most of the 422 alcoholics he studied were al-lergic to wheat or rye. Alcohol consumption causes and worsens abnormal intestinal permeability and is thought by many to be both the cause and effect of food allergies. Food-allergic and gluten-sensitive individuals often report more frequent and severe allergic reactions to foods in conjunction with alcohol consumption. Because of the genetic component in alcohol-ism, we suspect that the predisposition to alcoholism also predisposes to an abnormally permeable intestine and proneness to food sensitization.

Schizophrenia

Medical science took yet another leap forward when Dr. F. Dohan, a Philadelphia researcher and psychiatrist, learned that schizophrenia is frequently found in people with celiac disease, and celiac disease is frequently found in people with schizophrenia. He further found that in cultures where gluten-containing grains are rarely eaten, schizophrenia is rare or nonexistent. His dogged pursuit of this connection is the wellspring of a whole new understanding of diet-induced mental illness, and his work serves as a model for investigating other dietary ailments.

Unfortunately, schizophrenics are rarely tested for gluten sensitivity. A more recent report provides a startling example of this connection. A thirty-three-year-old man who was previously diagnosed with schizophrenia showed reduced blood flow to a frontal lobe of his brain. This is common in schizophrenia as well as in brain-sensitive food-allergic patients. This young man later developed some of the classic signs and symptoms of celiac disease, so he was tested. After he began a gluten-free diet, not only did his celiac symptoms disappear but also his symptoms of schizophrenia. Further, and perhaps more important, the pattern of blood flow in his brain also normalized.

This case, of course, is powerful support for Dohan's pioneering work in this area, but it is also vastly more than that. This one case connects compromised blood flow or blood vessel constriction in the context of schizophrenia and celiac disease. It also establishes gluten as the cause of this constriction by demonstrating that the constriction resolves on a gluten-free diet, and the patient recovers from both ailments.

This finding has implications for a range of ailments from strokes, to seizures, to autism, to aneurysms, to severe headaches. Migrainelike headaches are overrepresented in people with celiac disease and gluten sensitivity. Symptoms improve on a gluten-free diet, and celiac disease is overrepresented among those who chronically experience severe headaches.

Conventionally, ergotamine is the prescribed medication for the treatment of migraine headaches. Ergotamine causes constriction of blood vessels, thereby reducing the pain caused by vessel expansion in the brain of a migraineur. Eliminating allergic foods, including gluten, also can result in the elimination or lessening of migraine pain. Our position is that it is no accident that ergotamine is refined from a fungus that grows on gluten-rich rye and other grains.

Similarly, the hallucinogenic drug LSD is also derived from molds that grow on gluten grains. The hallucinations experienced in ergotamine poisoning may result from similar peptides gaining access to the brain. Some celiac patients undergoing a gluten challenge also experience hallucinations. Although there is not enough evidence to assert a connection, there is certainly enough to raise our suspicions about gluten as the common, underlying element in these conditions.

Taken together with gluten-derived exorphins, the impact of grains on schizophrenia seems evident and predictable. As a biochemical ailment, schizophrenia serves as an excellent reminder that psychiatric illness is just that—an illness. And many cases involve exorphins, peptides that cause blood vessel expansion and contraction, changes in neurotransmitter balance, and hallucinations.

EPILEPSY

Our case against gluten is particularly strong in the areas of gluten-induced epilepsy and disorders of blood vessels in the brain. Severe epileptic seizures, particularly those associated with calcium deposits in the brain; migraine headaches; and/or hyperactivity, often respond very well to a strict gluten-free diet. These improvements sometimes reduce or eliminate the need for antiseizure medications, even in cases where seizures had previously been poorly responsive to drug therapies.

In most cases of epilepsy, seizures can be lessened or eliminated with drugs, but about 20 to 30 percent of cases do not respond well to drugs. For some of these seizure victims, a diagnosis of celiac disease can have some very positive results.

Published reports of food allergy–induced seizures go all the way back to 1914. Although there were a few reports of the causative relationship between celiac disease and epilepsy prior to the late 1980s, the connection has received increasing attention over the last fifteen years or so. Celiac-associated epilepsy has been reported to occur in connection with migraine headaches, hyperactivity, calcium deposits in the brain, and in cases of blood vessel abnormalities in the brain. Celiac disease is now well recognized as a factor in most cases of epilepsy where calcium deposits are found in certain regions of the brain.

For some time, such connections were thought to be more than coincidence, but the issue was never investigated. Finally, in 1998, in a study where the prevailing rate of celiac disease was established at 1 in 244 pregnant women, celiac disease was found in 4 of 177 epileptic patients. That translates to a rate of 1 in 44 people with various forms of epilepsy who also have celiac disease. Judging from that research, celiac disease appears six times more frequently among those suffering from epilepsy. The occurrence of celiac disease is probably even greater among those with epilepsy associated with calcium deposits in the brain, although that question awaits further research.

Perhaps the most encouraging element of this connection between gluten and seizures is that some people with epilepsy find that their seizures stop after they begin the diet. Others report that their seizures are less frequent and easier to control with drugs when following a gluten-free diet. The evidence suggests that many individuals living with epilepsy would benefit from such a diet, regardless of their test results for gluten sensitivity. Unpredictable seizures and unpleasant side effects from antiseizure medications both seem a greater hardship than switching to a gluten-free diet.

AUTISM

Autism is another increasingly prevalent brain disorder where a strict gluten-free and dairy-free diet shows surprising, at times startling, improvements. The improvements were marked by better eye contact, less hyperactivity, enhanced verbal and cognitive skills, and greater sociability,

Symptoms of Autism Reversed
on a Gluten-Free Diet

My son first developed bowel problems as a small child subsequent to his immunizations. He was also constipated alternating with diarrhea. He descended into autism. He was unable to make controlled movements, a condition called apraxia. He was almost nonverbal. The speech therapist had to use sign language to work with him. This was at four years old. He had almost no speech and few appropriate play skills. He could spend up to eight hours a day switching lights off and on.

The school psychologist said that he belonged in a county-run preschool class. I observed the class and saw kids curled up in corners. They were low functioning with no apparent speech capability. The professionals said that with luck, by elementary school, my son would be in a special "autistic" class, possibly mainstreamed in one or two nonacademic areas. His future seemed very bleak.

I did some research on the Internet, then had my son tested for food allergies. He showed antibodies to dairy and gluten. I began removing gluten from his diet when he was between four and five years old. He has been strictly gluten free with only a few accidents. The results have been amazing. He went from being totally in his own world to being an engaged child. The cloud lifted.

Now, at nine, he is in a regular classroom, performing at grade level. He just won the school spelling bee, is on a baseball team, and is a competitive Irish dancer.

I am very glad I was able to access the Internet and read the works of Ron Hoggan, Ray Audette, and others.

Mary H.

in a substantial majority of cases, but the diet does not seem to completely cure the disorder.

Autistic children show strong evidence of delayed-onset IgG mediated food allergy, including recurrent middle-ear infections, epilepsy (one-third of autistics will suffer from seizures by adolescence), red ears, powerful food cravings, leaky gut, pronounced digestive problems, sleep disorders, hyperactivity, abnormal blood flow to certain areas of the brain, and many other conditions associated with gluten sensitivity.

Autism is another example of a condition where there is often no detectable celiac disease, but where gluten sensitivity plays a key role. Why, then, do many autistic children improve on a gluten-free, dairy-free diet? We think it has more to do with a complex interaction between digestive enzymes and intestinal permeability. Absorption of partly digested gluten and other foods, in combination with an abnormally permeable intestine, is an important part of this incomplete picture.

The successful but highly controversial use of an injectable form of synthetic secretin, a gut hormone, in the treatment of autistic children is another direction from which there is support for the role of a gluten-free diet. Research shows that secretin receptors are found not only in the intestinal tract, but the heart and brain tissues as well. Amazingly, the brain secretin appears to influence cognition, emotions, and behavior. Dietary gluten in an untreated celiac patient is a powerful inhibitor of secretin release, reducing blood levels of secretin by 90 percent. Eliminate gluten from the diet, and blood secretin levels return to near normal. A majority of autistic children experience improvements in cognition, behavior, emotions, verbal communication, and eye contact.

In another controversial study, Andrew Wakefield and his research team demonstrated that there is an increase in intestinal permeability, which may result from prior immunization in some autistic children. Such increased intestinal permeability suggests a path into the bloodstream for opioid and other peptides from partly digested gluten and dairy proteins.

A study by K. L. Reichelt and his colleagues reported abnormal quantities of urinary polypeptides in autistic children, which improved dramatically, along with similarly dramatic symptom improvement, on a gluten-free, dairy-free diet.

For some time now, measurements of urinary peptides have revealed that autistic, schizophrenic, and depressed patients excrete large quantities of peptides that can function as neurotransmitters. Such increases may be either a direct or an indirect result of leakage of exorphins into the bloodstream. This important clue to the cause of at least some cases of these psychiatric illnesses may indicate that these psychoactive peptides are small enough to be ignored by the immune system but function as potent neurotransmitters.

Autism-Gluten Connection

There is further evidence supporting the connection between gluten and autism. Paul Shattock, a plant biochemist and lecturer at the University of Sunderland, began collecting data and evaluating research when his son was diagnosed with autism in 1974. When he heard speculation that autism may be the result of peptide poisoning, he began investigating the possibility that gluten and dairy were at the root of his son's condition. Similarly, Kalle Reichelt, a researcher at the Pediatric Research Institute in Oslo, Norway, also became interested in the possibility that peptides from gluten and dairy products contribute to autism in his patients. By 1990, Reichelt and Shattock had learned through their own investigations that 90 percent of the autistic patients they studied have abnormally high levels of urinary peptides. The evidence suggests that these peptides are from dairy products and gluten cereals.

This research, in conjunction with earlier work by Dohan, has established a connection between gluten consumption and several types of mental illnesses, behavioral problems, and learning disabilities. However, broader recognition of these discoveries is slow.

Concerned parents and others may want to act more quickly on this information, as the appropriate diet is very safe and nutritious. Other than the inconvenience of implementing the diet while ensuring optimal nutrition, there is no known downside to this therapy. Those who currently struggle with these conditions will be unlikely to benefit from this information if they await its general acceptance before changing their diet.

MULTIPLE SCLEROSIS (MS) AND GLUTEN

A degenerative disease of the central nervous system, MS is another condition where improvements have repeatedly been reported after beginning a gluten-free diet. It is a condition that is characterized by damage resulting from the immune system's attack on the fatty coating on nerves, called myelin, which serve as insulation for nerves. This insulation allows the speedy passage of impulses along nerves. Without myelin, the neurological dysfunction of MS soon follows, resulting in symptoms that include chronic fatigue, loss of balance, clumsiness, reduced vision, bouts of localized paralysis, bladder problems, muscle spasticity, weakness, numbness, depression, and intellectual changes. The famous British playwright Roger MacDougall reported his own amazing recovery from a terribly disabling form of MS. Although he experienced a remission, not a cure, his improvement was nothing short of miraculous.

How did he do it? As a result of his reading and research, Professor MacDougall reasoned that his condition was the result of a chemical imbalance and that his best hope was to eat a diet that probably shaped human evolution. He cleverly decided to follow a diet that closely paralleled that of a prehistoric hunter-gatherer—one that excluded dairy and gluten. MacDougall not only experienced a dramatic recovery but also went on to write about his recovery and the means by which he achieved it in a pamphlet published by Regenics, Inc., a vitamin company with offices in the United Kingdom and United States.

Four years after his own diagnosis of multiple sclerosis, Scottish biochemist Norman Matheson, Ph.D., was inspired by MacDougall. Although not as debilitated as MacDougall, Dr. Matheson experienced a speedy recovery as a result of a gluten-free diet. His report appeared in the October 5, 1974, issue of *Lancet*.

Although in his declining years Matheson questioned the utility of the

Gluten-Causing Symptoms of MS

A few years ago I found myself faced with what doctors suspected were a growing number of symptoms of multiple sclerosis. I was experiencing extreme muscular, neurological, cognitive, and gait abnormalities.

With some encouragement from a friend and support from family, I found my way to a Paleolithic diet. I tried it with a "nothing to lose" attitude. To my surprise, my symptoms began to fade within the first few weeks.

Through trial and error, I've found it was processed foods that had caused my health to be greatly compromised. Foods containing gluten cause the most severe reaction. Within a few hours of an accidental ingestion, symptoms return. I then have a minimum recovery period of a week before symptoms subside.

It wasn't what I needed to add to my diet, but rather what I needed to delete (all processed foods) that was key to my recovery.

Patti V.

diet, his astuteness and alert demeanor would be considered a blessing to any elderly MS patient fortunate enough to live so long with the disease.

Still, we do realize that the evidence only supports dietary intervention in some MS patients. We also acknowledge that other factors may play key roles in MS, including excessive oxidative stress from vitamin E, glutathione, CoQ_{10} deficiencies, and increased intestinal permeability. To our knowledge, only one group has investigated intestinal permeability in MS. They found that 25 percent of the MS patients they investigated had increased intestinal permeability. This increase may simply allow gluten proteins to leak into the bloodstream. As we established in an earlier chapter, these proteins have been shown to injure a variety of human tissues. However, it is a likely possibility that partial or whole proteins from gluten are leaked into the bloodstream and that they trigger an inappropriate attack by the immune system on the MS patient's myelin.

CONCLUSION

There are many brain and nerve disorders that can be impacted by eating gluten. A great deal of research is needed to clarify the role that gluten plays in these ailments. Much of it will have to wait for at least another decade as knowledge of the health hazards of gluten becomes more widespread. In the meantime, readers of this book who are challenged by gluten-induced brain and nerve diseases will have to find their own way through the labyrinth of confusion surrounding these conditions, hopefully linking with other like-minded individuals who recognize the importance of diet in these conditions.

Bowel Diseases
and Gluten

Many people incorrectly assume that gluten sensitivity is a bowel disease. The bowel is certainly where suggestive symptoms and confirming evidence of celiac disease were first identified. However, gluten sensitivity and celiac disease usually affect the entire body. Because the bowel's dual, and somewhat contradictory, function of protecting us from the environment while it absorbs nutrients from that same environment is a complex task that is fraught with hazards, there is certainly a bowel component to the disease. The bowel is where susceptible individuals allow the different gluten proteins into their circulation, but the impact of these proteins may manifest in any organ or body system.

We consider it a fundamental mistake to limit our understanding of gluten sensitivity by labeling it as a bowel disease. But there is considerable room for confusion on this issue.

It Took Forty Years to Diagnose

I am seventy-two years old. Somewhere around the time of bearing children, I developed severe constipation. It ruled my life for the last forty years. I suffered from occasional impactions, lots of foul-smelling gas, lots of discomfort, etc. I changed doctors several times, and everyone, including my present gastroenterologist, diagnosed me with Irritable Bowel Syndrome (IBS). I even participated in a study on a drug for IBS that resulted in my being hospitalized for nine days.

About two years ago, no matter what or how much I ate, I couldn't keep on the weight. At that time I developed occasional bouts of diarrhea mixed with the severe constipation. I had very occasional episodes of nausea and vomiting, but each time we thought it was food poisoning or the stomach flu. I became so weak that I was homebound, and the doctor did countless tests. I think he was looking for cancer. After about four months of testing, the final resort was random biopsies of my small intestine. Guess what? I had flattened villi.

Within days of going gluten free, I felt well and have been well ever since. Although the constipation has not completely resolved, twice daily ingestions of Metamucil keep things moving, and I am back traveling and living a normal life. In the last few months, my daughter, my son, and my brother have all had positive blood tests. My seventy-year-old brother even had a positive biopsy, but his gastroenterologist told him that with no symptoms, at his age, he can ignore it. My daughter had stomach problems and was biopsy diagnosed and is now healthy and gluten free.

Renee C.

IRRITABLE BOWEL SYNDROME (IBS)

First, let's look at irritable bowel syndrome, or IBS. Although people with IBS may look normal and healthy, they suffer from chronic stomach cramps or pain, diarrhea alternating with constipation and bloating, and many psychological symptoms. It is the most common bowel disease in the industrial world, afflicting about 22 percent of the Western population, conservatively estimated at about 85 million people. Dr. Joseph Murray of the Mayo Clinic in Rochester, Minnesota, has presented data showing that about half of those with untreated celiac disease fit the diagnostic criteria for IBS, known as the ROME criteria. That means that in the absence of blood tests and/or intestinal biopsy, we can expect that many people with celiac disease currently have a diagnosis of IBS.

These findings are reflected in other research. One group of researchers found that 12 percent of the group of IBS patients they studied actually had celiac disease when they were tested for it. Another group reported that 20 percent of their IBS patients suffer from celiac disease. Think that one over for a moment. These studies indicate that anywhere from 10.2 to 17 million people are likely to have undetected celiac disease. Such reports indicate that a very significant minority of the people suffering from IBS would greatly benefit from a gluten-free diet.

Non-celiac gluten sensitivity is much more common than celiac disease. Therefore, many, perhaps most, patients with IBS who do not have biopsy-provable celiac disease may still be gluten sensitive and would benefit from a gluten-free diet. Like all deductions, our conclusion is only a reasonable probability until it is tested. However, the clues and evidence are quite persuasive.

Although they may share common symptoms, we make a clear distinction between celiac disease and IBS. Often poorly understood, IBS is also poorly defined and is usually diagnosed through the exclusion of other diseases. IBS frequently responds poorly to conventional medical therapies. On the other hand, there is a clear, well-established diagnostic protocol and very effective treatment for celiac disease.

A gluten-free diet has often been found to alleviate some or all of the symptoms of IBS. For example, it has been reported that up to 70 percent of all IBS patients improve with food exclusion. The majority improve with the individual elimination of wheat, and many others benefit from exclusion of oats and rye. We can only surmise that exclusion of all gluten grains would be a valuable therapy for most of these patients.

Percentage of 122 IBS Patients Intolerant to Glutens and Other Foods

CEREALS	FRUIT	VEGETABLES	DAIRY	MEAT	MISCELLANEOUS
wheat 60%	citrus 24%	onions 22%	cow's milk 44%	beef 16%	coffee 33%
corn 44%	apples 12%	potatoes 20%	cheese 39%	pork 14%	eggs 26%
oats 34%		cabbage 19%	butter 25%	chicken 13%	tea 25%
rye 30%		sprouts 18%	yogurt 21%	lamb 11%	chocolate 22%
barley 24%		peas 17%			nuts 22%
rice 15%		carrots 15%			

Hunter, J.O., et al. "Dietary studies." In *Topics in gastroenterology 12*, ed. P. R. Gibson and D. P. Jewell (Oxford: Blackwell Scientific, 1985), pp. 305–13.

Why, you might ask, in the face of such evidence, would the potential therapeutic value of a gluten-free diet be ignored? The answer is simple: Celiac disease is defined by biopsy-proven damage to the lining. Such damage is not found in about 80 percent of people with IBS, so a gluten-free diet is not yet considered an appropriate therapy for most cases of IBS. A majority of 85 million IBS sufferers are condemned to a life of discomfort as a result of this narrow, outdated definition of gluten sensitivity. We recommend IgG and IgA anti-gliadin and EMA or tTG antibody screening of all patients with IBS. Positive test results should lead to a prescription of a gluten-free diet.

INTESTINAL INFECTIONS, FOOD ALLERGY, AND GLUTEN SENSITIVITY

Intestinal infection is another range of ailments where we recommend antibody testing and a trial of a gluten-free diet. Gluten sensitivity is often a contributing factor in chronic diarrhea, even where infection is the primary problem. It also makes sense to consider antibody testing since those with untreated celiac disease are also at greater risk of contracting infectious diseases.

For patients with chronic diarrhea that is poorly responsive to conventional therapies, it makes perfect sense to consider IgG ELISA delayed food allergy, IgG and IgA anti-gliadin, and EMA or tTG celiac screening tests.

CROHN'S DISEASE

Crohn's disease is somewhat different from celiac disease, although both conditions share many symptoms and features. Crohn's disease is an inflammation of the full thickness of the bowel wall and may impact on any part of the GI tract, from mouth to anus. The inflammatory injuries in celiac disease, on the other hand, are restricted to the thin mucosal lining of the digestive tract and do not usually penetrate all layers of the bowel wall. In Crohn's disease, however, patients develop openings in the bowel wall, called fistulas, that actually allow the bowel contents to take shortcuts between different parts of the small intestine. This results in parts of the bowel where there is little or no movement of the contents. It doesn't take much of an imagination to appreciate how infectious and painful the areas that are isolated by fistulas can become.

Gluten-induced injury to the bowel wall is the primary, defining characteristic of celiac disease. But these injuries do not usually penetrate all layers of the bowel wall. These distinctions become less clear with increased attention to detail, but the general principle does differentiate the two diseases. Does that mean that Crohn's patients would not benefit from a gluten-free diet? The evidence suggests otherwise.

Crohn's patients have very high levels of antibodies against gliadin proteins, indicating a leaky gut, an immune response, and sensitivity to gluten. Yet, due to a failure to recognize non-celiac gluten sensitivity, conventional medical wisdom ignores positive blood tests and gluten's contribution to the pain suffered by these people. Crohn's patients may hear advice suggesting that they avoid foods that bother them, but that is very different than encouraging patients to follow a strict gluten-free diet for several months or a lifetime. Silent celiac disease and delayed reaction to food allergens can result in most people being unaware of which foods are problematic. Many Crohn's patients may not know that they have quite elevated levels of gliadin antibodies and therefore should avoid gluten.

Due to the difficulty in self-diagnosing food sensitivities, testing for IgG and IgA anti gliadin antibodies and for IgG delayed-type food sensitivities is probably the best approach to determining which foods should be eliminated from a Crohn's patient's diet. Another alternative is to recommend that Crohn's patients keep a symptom and food diary to monitor any changes. Although much less accurate than blood testing, these tools may prove helpful to some. Testing for the presence of antibodies to foods or food components is by far the preferable alternative in this situation.

ENTERITIS, FOOD ALLERGY, AND GLUTEN SENSITIVITY

We have already discussed the benefits of a gluten-free, dairy-free diet for those who develop inflammation of the small intestines, called enteritis, as a result of cancer treatments. We suspect that similar benefits might accrue to some patients who suffer from bacterial and viral enteritis.

Regardless of the cause of bowel disease, we recommend a gluten-free, dairy-free diet in addition to other restorative therapies.

SWOLLEN LYMPH GLANDS AND GLUTEN

On physical examination some celiac patients appear to have developed a malignant mass in their small intestine. A more discriminating investigation sometimes reveals that excessively swollen lymph nodes are the problem. The swelling recedes on a gluten-free diet.

MICROSCOPIC AND ULCERATIVE COLITIS

There is considerable genetic overlap between celiac disease and an inflammation of the colon, called microscopic colitis, and patients often reflect this association in their symptoms. If you suffer from colitis and it is not getting any better, you may also have to deal with the complication of celiac disease. Celiacs are similarly at high risk of developing microscopic colitis.

In addition to the symptoms, there are frequently elevated levels of IgG and/or IgA gliadin antibodies in colitis patients. This strongly suggests that gluten is a contributing factor in the signs and symptoms of colitis.

TAKING A POSITION ON GUT DISEASE

Given the evidence, we argue that treatment of any medical condition connected with a leaky or malabsorbing gut ought to automatically include a food allergy–gluten-sensitivity workup, possibly leading to a recommendation of a gluten-free/food allergy–free diet. Beyond intestinal diseases, conditions associated with a leaky or flat gut include a variety of liver diseases, pancreatic diseases, and several eating disorders. Of course, we make the same recommendation for autoimmune diseases, along with a host of other chronic conditions where the laboratory evidence points directly to gluten as a factor in the disease process.

Do not misunderstand. It is far from clear whether gluten actually causes the underlying disease, but it is very clear that exclusion of gluten is likely to provide some degree of relief from many bowel symptoms. By excluding gluten, many patients may be able to stop the escalating cycle of increased intestinal permeability, leakage of gluten into the blood-

Gut Symptoms that Can Be Alleviated by a Gluten-Free Diet

1. abdominal pain
2. chronic diarrhea of unknown cause
3. steatorhea (excessive fat in stools)
4. recurrent aphthous ulcers (multiple, painful canker sores)
5. nausea and vomiting
6. bloating, abdominal distention
7. flatulence
8. GI bleeding (often X-ray negative)
9. angular stomatitis
10. glossitis, macroglossia (enlarged, inflamed tongue)
11. gastric and duodenal ulcers (in patients unresponsive to conventional antibiotic therapies for *Helicobacter pylori*)
12. abnormal intestinal permeability (leaky gut)
13. pancreatic insufficiency
14. gut hormone inhibition (secretin and cholecystokinin, e.g.)
15. dyspepsia, esophageal reflux (5 percent of all such patients have gluten-induced loss of small intestinal lining = duodenal villous atrophy)

stream, increased antibody production, increased tissue damage, increased intestinal permeability, and increased need for symptom-chasing prescription medications.

Not surprisingly, all of the above symptoms are also common in celiac disease. The point is simple. We are not genetically well equipped to consume these grains.

Where to from Here? Research, Theories, and Treatments

Many of the theories related to gluten sensitivity and celiac disease are still in their infancy, early adolescence at best. This is in large part the result of the popular belief, perpetuated with the very best of intentions by cereal manufacturers, dietitians, and the USDA food pyramid, that gluten cereals are very healthy, wholesome foods for the masses. If it is true that the slow advancement in gluten research is the result of the scarcity of research funding, it is doubly true that many health professionals are not taking time to keep up with the mountain of published research in this area.

In spite of an inevitable resistance to new ideas, research into the health hazards of gluten cereals is becoming a dominant force. This very good news can only lead to promising discoveries that will improve patient care as well as point the direction for future research.

On the other hand, as in any area of innovation, there are also mistaken beliefs that persist or even gain support. The notion that "celiac disease is rare" is a classic example of this. Mistaken ideas risk poorer patient care and increase human suffering.

Nevertheless, the current state of gluten research is overwhelmingly positive, favoring rapid progress and improved patient care. Indeed, these are good times.

Celiac disease, as a subset of gluten sensitivity, has received the most research attention. Because there is a great deal more information about celiac disease than other expressions of gluten sensitivity, it provides the best window through which to examine most areas of gluten sensitivity and, hence, the best starting point for discussing variations in gluten sensitivity.

PROGRESS IS NOT SIMPLE OR EASY

At least on the surface, expansion of human knowledge in a given field appears to be a linear progression moving from one advancement to the next, ever increasing and broadening our understanding. However, a closer look reveals that the growth of knowledge has never been that simple or easy. Advances in gluten-sensitivity research are always punctuated by interminable delays and innocent errors stacked on top of lingering misconceptions.

If we expect to see the same clear, straightforward progress in gluten research that accompanies more developed fields, such as surgery or trauma care, we will be disappointed.

Nevertheless, new advancements and possibilities are happening right now. Let's take a closer look.

FUTURE GLUTEN RESEARCH

Several areas of gluten research show great promise. For the last four decades or so, the overriding belief has been that only gliadins in the gluten protein, the peptides that cause villous atrophy, are harmful. Therefore, the other peptides that make up gluten, such as the glutenins, are interesting, perhaps, but basically harmless. Current research is beginning to refute this notion.

Glutenin

Van de Wal and colleagues have identified a glutenin peptide that activates T-lymphocyte immune cells in the small intestine in much the same way as gliadin, suggesting that glutenin may also be involved in the disease process. In addition, glutenin seems to cross-react with elastin, the principal component of elastic tissues, suggesting that glutenin may play a role in autoimmune diseases of the skin. Other studies indicate that glutenin peptides are toxic to cells. Even worse news for those gluten-sensitive people who turn to rice as a dietary refuge, glutenin antibodies appear to cross-react with rice, perhaps placing rice off-limits to many glutenin-sensitive people.

Clearly, gliadin is not the only toxic component of gluten, and blood tests that exclusively identify antibodies sensitized to gliadin appear to be inadequate for identifying everyone who is gluten sensitive. Innovative laboratories are currently developing a new IgG and IgA anti-glutenin immunoassay to compliment the anti-gliadin test, which should be available sometime in 2002. We would encourage research into sensitivity to the other gluten peptides, such as globulin and albumin.

Another approach would involve exposing blood drawn from treated celiacs to similarly purified gluten. The absence of an immune reaction would certainly support the notion that only the identified peptides are harmful. We are skeptical. We suspect that we still have a great deal to learn in this area and that there are many harmful proteins to be found in gluten grains. Only further research will tell.

Issues that Should Shape New Research Designs

When a celiac patient is consuming a gluten-free diet, a gluten challenge often involves very large quantities of gluten over a fairly lengthy period, sometimes years, before the intestinal biopsy will reveal the anticipated gluten-induced damage. Clearly, the intestinal biopsy is not a highly sensitive procedure that will always detect small quantities of gluten in the diet. Yet, this is the test that usually serves as the basis for the rationale used to justify the unfortunate practice of recommending consumption of malt-flavored breakfast cereals and a general disregard for small quantities of gluten in the diet. Negative endomysium antibody tests are also used to justify the recommendation of these foods to celiac patients. As we have established previously, these tests are least sensitive to cases where the intestinal damage is less severe. The use of these tests to support these recommendations is illogical.

Such recommendations may lead hospital staff to serve such foods to celiac patients in the belief that it does no harm. Dietitians and gastroenterologists sometimes use the same faulty reasoning to recommend such foods to celiac patients. We suspect that these recommendations are rooted in the perspective that the gluten-free diet is unpleasant and that this more liberal approach is considered more humane.

PROBLEMS WITH CURRENT RESEARCH METHODS

We also need to develop some new methods for conducting this research.

Placebo Effect

Because our minds can sometimes play tricks on us, researchers have had to develop ways of telling whether a particular drug or therapy caused subjects to experience improvements in whatever condition was being studied or whether the subjects were reporting changes because of the psychological impact of the research program.

Double-Blind Crossover

The research method that has gained the widest acceptance is called the double-blind crossover design. This approach does not allow either the subjects or those administering the drug to know whether individual subjects are receiving the placebo or the active drug. If the research requires that subjects be observed or tested, those performing the observations or conducting the tests must also be unaware of the grouping of research subjects and the treatment they have been given. The researchers and subjects are both said to be "blind."

The crossover part of the design requires that subjects experience some exposure to both the placebo and the drug. For part of the experiment, a given subject will receive the placebo. For another segment of the experiment, the same subject will receive the drug. There is often a wash-out period when neither the drug nor the placebo is taken. This is done to ensure that the drug has been eliminated from the subject's system. Responses during each period are recorded and then tabulated. The placebo effect, where subjects report anticipated changes, can be reported along with fairly accurate indications of the drug's effectiveness.

New Designs Needed for Dietary Interventions

Such approaches as the double-blind, crossover design are not well suited to investigating dietary interventions. This is true for several reasons. It is difficult to mask the taste and texture of foods. The presence or absence of gluten is very difficult to mask. Dohan et al. answered this problem by placing all the inmates on a locked psychiatric ward on a gluten-free, dairy-free diet. Both groups were also given a daily beverage. One contained gluten, while the other did not. Unfortunately, this required that many of the hospital personnel be aware of which beverage contained the gluten, so the design was not double-blind.

Further, most dietary intervention research cannot reasonably include the incarceration of their human subjects in a locked facility.

There are some reports of research where containment on a locked ward was already in place, but this feature was undermined by the practice of allowing visitors to bring food to patients during the experiment. This work clearly shows some of the difficulty with dietary research.

Because of the general perception of the harmlessness of foods derived from gluten and dairy products, it is also difficult to control for outside contamination by staff members. Without appropriate support, the generosity of staff and visitors threatens the integrity of dietary research, even on a locked ward. When the aid of these individuals is enlisted, the research design may be compromised if we adhere to the design that was developed for testing drug interventions.

Another problem with the use of a double-blind, crossover approach is that the impact of dietary substances is often delayed. This can result in delayed improvements that show up during the placebo phase and failure to improve during the intervention. It is confounding results such as these that undermine dietary research yet are the predictable result of using research methods that were designed for, and are well suited to, pharmaceutical research. Appropriate experimental designs for dietary interventions are needed.

Symptom Chasing or Treating the Cause

Another factor in this mix is that advances in drug research continue to provide increasingly sophisticated chemical tools for masking symptoms and manipulating body chemistry rather than pursuing underlying causes of symptoms. Considerable expenditure of talent, time, and money for symptom chasing invariably reduces available resources for the search for underlying causes.

NEW PERSPECTIVES AND PARADIGM SHIFTS

Many encouraging perspectives and exciting areas of research have moved to the forefront among prominent researchers. As these new perspectives are studied, new ways of thinking about and understanding celiac disease and gluten sensitivity will develop.

Gluten and Viruses

One avenue of research is driven by the notion that celiac disease not only needs the genetic predisposition but also requires the exposure to particular viruses before it can develop. Antibodies against adenovirus 12, for instance, are found much more commonly among those with celiac disease. Gluten-induced illnesses, such as insulin-dependent diabetes, may also be a case in point, where infectious agents have started the disease process by causing a leaky gut and, hence, contamination of the bloodstream with food proteins and peptides.

Gluten and Germs

The germ theory, first postulated more than 150 years ago, suggested that disease is caused by invisible atomies, which we now call microbes. This theory, coupled with advances in surgical intervention, has driven most medical research during the last century. These advances, along with improved sanitation, a more abundant food supply, and an infrastructure that permits rapid treatment of traumatic injuries, have all combined to extend longevity. These are venerable achievements. However, the paradigm that was shaped by these theories and advances has also slowed and misdirected research related to cancer, osteoporosis, autoimmunity, some types of brain disease, celiac disease, and many types of bowel disease.

In other words, the current way of thinking is not only shaped by the germ theory, it appears inconsistent with many of the imperatives of dietary diseases such as gluten sensitivity and celiac disease. For example, despite compelling research to the contrary, whole-gluten cereals are still touted as a healthy food by many medical doctors, most certified dietitians, and many health-food stores. This, of course, is changing, but much too slowly. The unfortunate truth is that, at a time when literally tens of thousands of published studies are indicating the medicinal value of diet and nutrition, inadequate dietary instruction is being offered to physicians and dietitians. Both groups continue to be swayed by outdated perspectives, allopathic prejudices, NIH pronouncements, and the Department of Agriculture's promotional literature, especially the infamous food pyramid.

Reversal and Prevention of Autoimmune Disease on a Gluten-Free Diet?

Studies involving lab animals genetically prone to insulin-dependent diabetes (IDDM) when eating diabetogenic foods such as gluten cereals have shown that, in advance of the clinical expression of IDDM, there is insulin cell inflammation and elevation of blood levels of anti-gluten IgG or IgA antibodies, indicating a slow but inexorable progression toward the clinical disease. With the elimination of the gluten cereals that are provoking an immune response, the progression toward clinical IDDM abates. This indicates that, with early detection and dietary change, IDDM can be prevented and possibly avoided indefinitely. Human studies involving siblings of diagnosed diabetic children are currently under way to test this extraordinarily provocative hypothesis.

Similarly, a recent study involving patients with celiac disease and autoimmune thyroid disease indicates that early detection of gluten sensitivity and gluten elimination not only causes anti-gliadin antibodies to disappear, but thyroid-specific autoantibodies as well. This may not only help to reverse autoimmune thyroid disease but also prevent the development of other gluten-associated autoimmune diseases.

Glutamine for Villous Atrophy and a Leaky Gut

L-glutamine, the most abundant amino acid in the blood, brain, and skeletal muscle, is a tasteless, nontoxic, conditionally essential amino acid that appears to be showing promise in the treatment of celiac disease. Research demonstrates that glutamine is the primary fuel for the lining of the small intestine and immune system.

When given in therapeutic doses (9–20 grams a day in divided doses), it also releases growth hormone and increases the production of a powerful, detoxifying, antioxidant enzyme called glutathione peroxidase. Glutamine also seems to protect the intestinal lining from the destructive action of alcohol, NSAIDS, and aspirin. It has been reported that glutamine is now the most popular anti-ulcer medication in Asia because it heals and helps prevent peptic ulcers. In a recent study in Japan, 92 percent of ulcer patients given 1,600 milligrams of glutamine a day showed complete healing of duodenal and peptic ulcers in four weeks. It is also currently being administered intravenously to patients receiving major abdominal and bone marrow surgery, therapy for third-degree burns, and chemotherapy or radiation therapy for cancer.

From our perspective, the single most promising benefit of glutamine is that, when removed from the diet, it may prevent and reverse villous atrophy, a leaky gut, and the malabsorption of nutrients so commonly seen in celiac disease and Crohn's disease.

We would conjecture that glutamine's primary value will not be to substitute a gluten-free diet, but to help accelerate healing when initially going off gluten and to lessen intestinal inflammation when gluten is inadvertently or intentionally reintroduced back into the diet.

There are many such murky issues in the infant field of immune reactions to grain proteins. Each issue warrants appropriate research, which will translate into health benefits for many.

Population Screening

Another new perspective, beginning with a general recognition that celiac disease is a common but badly underestimated condition, has led to recommendations that screening for celiac disease be performed in all six-year-old children, regardless if symptomatic, in entire school districts in Italy.

Italy is at the forefront of research in the area of population screening. Italian researchers are now conducting AGA blood testing on all beginning students of entire school districts. Those who show IgG and/or IgA anti-gliadin antibodies are then tested for the presence of endomysium antibodies. Where parents give their permission, if the EMA comes back positive, an endoscopy is conducted to look for the characteristic intestinal damage of celiac disease.

The first stage of this research first revealed that celiac disease was not rare, even in a country that is relatively close to the Fertile Crescent and where gluten forms a large part of many traditional foods. The startling rates found in Italy were the first step toward recognizing that populations further removed from the Fertile Crescent would demonstrate even higher rates of celiac disease.

We highly recommend the same screening program for Canada and the United States—but with one caveat: Italian researchers are currently focused on finding, diagnosing, and treating only celiac disease. While we have great admiration for the exciting work they are doing in identifying those with celiac disease, we would respectfully recommend a gluten-free diet to all children who have non-celiac gluten sensitivity.

Such population screening and recommendations will predictably result in improved health and longevity for all of the gluten-sensitive individuals who are identified by this work and follow the appropriate treatment.

We look forward to the day when gluten-sensitivity testing will become routine. The time is rapidly approaching when you will be able to determine your own gluten and food-allergy status in the privacy of your own home with a simple self-administered, results-while-you-wait fingerstick. One or two drops of blood from your fingertip and within thirty minutes you will have accurate information regarding your sensitivity to gluten, gliadin, glutenin, wheat, and oats, along with common food allergens such as milk, soy, yeast, and eggs.

England-based York Nutritional Laboratories is currently researching and developing this innovative technology and hopes to make it commercially available to health consumers in Britain, Canada, and the United States sometime in 2002.

Screening for Additional Food Allergies

Frequently, a celiac patient, although improved on a gluten-free diet, will still experience chronic symptoms and illness. Recent clinical research suggests that additional delayed-onset food allergies coexist with celiac disease. When these allergens are eliminated from the diet, the residual symptoms disappear.

Yet, currently, such food allergies are rarely sought. Again, this reflects a perspective that is slowly surrendering to the growing body of evidence in support of food-allergy testing and health benefits that derive from it.

But there is a long way to go. Desensitization therapies are still offered, steroids are still considered a reasonable alternative to the gluten-free diet, and dapsone continues to be offered as an alternative to the gluten-free lifestyle. These perspectives, although waning, have some dangerous and deadly implications.

Understanding the Benefits of a Gluten-Free Diet

We have often heard about how unpalatable the gluten-free diet is. But we hear it from people who have never followed the diet. We suspect this says more about the speaker than about the gluten-free experience. Our own experiences argue the contrary prospective. We find the diet not only healthful but also enjoyable and fulfilling. The faulty assumption that excluding gluten is tantamount to deprivation, causing suffering, is foolish and limited. It may also reflect the addictive impact that this food can have on some individuals. More emphasis on educating the gluten-sensitive individual about the wide variety of palatable, tasty, gluten-free alternatives and integration of knowledge from the new medical specialty of addictionology are imperative.

New developments in screening and diagnostic tests should result in improved rates of diagnosis and improved treatments. Many of us will benefit from such advances.

Expanding Alternatives

Hopefully, advances in research may also occur in the area of farming and food production. At a time when more gluten is viewed as superior and highly desirable, pioneering work is currently aimed at developing a genetic strain of wheat that is free of the gluten proteins identified as harmful to celiacs. (Not surprisingly, genetically modified milk cows that can produce casein-free milk are also under research development.) Only time, effort, and money will tell whether or not the bakers and wheat-loving consumers will embrace these new hybrids.

Some grains such as rice, amaranth, and quinoa are relatively hypo-allergenic, so cutting-edge farmers, anticipating the trend, are slowly converting to non-gluten cereal grain production. As always, the health consumers, voting with their dollars, will persuade the farmers, General Mills and Post breakfast cereal companies, and the Department of Agriculture to accelerate this encouraging trend. We also anticipate that advancing gluten research will encourage farmers and manufacturers to produce and develop more gluten-free alternatives and hope that many of these changes will result in the cultivation and marketing of foodstuffs that are more consistent with our genetic heritage.

STAYING IN TOUCH

Much is happening in gluten research and clinical nutrition. Promising new studies and ideas abound. Some of the ideas in this book will be replaced by new insights as our understanding in this area expands. We would sincerely like to share with you these new findings and concepts as they appear, along with our interpretation and spin. You can stay in touch through our web sites www.cerealkillers.com (Braly) and www.dangerousgrains.com (Hoggan).

Common Signs and Symptoms of Celiac Disease

Alopecia

Anemias, especially iron and folic acid

Anorexia

Autism

Autoimmune arthritis

Autoimmune connective tissue diseases

Autoimmune thyroiditis

Cerebellar ataxia

Cerebral and cerebellar atrophy

Cerebral calcifications

Chromosome aberrations

Chronic fatigue

Chronic liver disease

Colitis

Constipation

Delayed puberty

Dental enamel defects

Depression

Down syndrome

Early menopause

Febrile seizures

Gallbladder dysfunction

Gallstones

Idiopathic thrombocytopenic purpura

IgA deficiency

IgA nephropath infertility

Insulin-dependent diabetes mellitus

Intestinal cancers

Kidney stones

Linear IgA dermatosis

Low calcium

Low iron

Low magnesium

Low vitamin A

Low vitamin D

Low vitamin K

Low zinc

Mild ataxia

Monoarthritis

Muscular hypotonia

Neurological disorders

Obesity

Obstructive pulmonary disease

Osteomalacia

Osteoporosis

Pancreatic insufficiency

Pica

Pulmonary bleeding

Retarded motor development

Rickets

Sacroileitis

Schizophrenia

Short stature

Single generalized seizures

Spontaneous, low-impact
   fractures

Systemic lupus erythematosus

White-matter brain lesions

Hidden Sources of Gluten

SAFE SOURCES AND INGREDIENTS IN FLOUR

Caveat: Always double-check for risk of contamination.

Acacia gum	Buckwheat	Flax
Alfalfa	Canola oil	Fruit
Algae	Carob flour	Gelatin
Almond	Cassava	Guar gum
Amaranth	Cellulose	Herbs
Arabic gum	Cellulose gum	Maize
Arrowroot	Chickpea	Maltodextrin
Artichokes	Corn	Methyl cellulose
Bean, adzuki	Corn flour	Millet
Bean, hyacinth	Cornmeal	Milo
Bean, lentil	Cornstarch	Nuts
Bean, mung	Corn syrup	Pea flour
Bean romano (chickpea)	Flaked rice	Peas

Potatoes

Potato flour

Psyllium

Quinoa

Rape

Rice

Rice flour

Seaweed

Sesame seed

Sorghum

Sorghum flour

Soy

Soybean

Spices

Sunflower seed

Sweet chestnut flour

Tapioca

Tapioca flour

Teff flour

Waxy maize

Whey

Wild rice

Xanthan gum

Yam flour

UNSAFE SOURCES OF FLOUR—MAY CONTAIN GLUTEN

Abyssinian hard
  wheat

Baking powder

Barley grass

Barley hordeum
  vulgare

Barley malt

Beer

Bleached flour

Blue cheese

Bran

Bread flour

Brewer's yeast

Brown flour

Bulgar

Bulgar wheat

Cereal binding

Chilton

Couscous

Dextrins

Durum wheat triticum

Edible starch

Einkorn wheat

Farina graham

Germ

Graham flour

Granary flour

Groats

Gum base

Hard wheat

Kamut

Malt

Matzo semolina

Miso

Mononoccum

Mustard powder

Oats

Oat straw

Pearl barley

Rice malt

Rye

Seitan

Semolina

Semolina triticum

Shoyu

Small spelt

Soba noodles

Soy sauce

Spelt

Sprouted wheat or barley

Stock cubes

Strong flour

Suet in packets

Tabbouleh

Teriyaki sauce

Triticale

Triticum aestivum

Triticum durum

Wheat nuts

Wheat triticum

Wheat germ oil

Wheat grass

Wheat starch

Adapted from http://www.celiac.com

ACRONYMS THAT MIGHT SPELL "HIDDEN" GLUTEN

Fu—dried wheat gluten

HPP—hydrolyzed plant protein

HVP—hydrolyzed vegetable protein

MSG—monosodium glutamate

TPP—textured plant protein

TVP—textured vegetable protein

Autoimmune Diseases Frequently Found in Celiac Disease

Alopecia areata

Arthritis

Atresia

Autoimmune thyroid disease

Biliary sclerosis

Cirrhosis

Crohn's disease

Diabetes mellitus

Fibromyalgia

Hypoparathyroidism

Idiopathic thrombocytopenic purpura

Microscopic colitis

Multiple sclerosis

Nephropathy (kidney disease)

Optic neuritis

Oral cankers

Sarcoidosis

Systemic lupus erythematosus

Trigeminal neuritis

Vasculitis

Comprehensive List
of Gluten-Associated
Medical Conditions

1. Abdominal distension/bloating
2. Abortions recurrent (15 percent of conceptions in patients with celiac disease end in miscarriages vs. 6 percent of controls)
3. Adenovirus gastroenteritis (may be triggered in latent celiac disease that initiates small bowel mucosal pathology)
4. Addison's disease (see Autoimmune diseases below)
5. AIDS (progression reflected by anti-gliadin Ab levels)
6. Albumin and prealbumin, serum (both low in CD)
7. Alkaline phosphatase, serum and bone (both elevated in CD)
8. Alopecia areata (both patchy and universal prevalence may be as high as 1 out of 85 celiacs, almost 3,000 times higher than predicted)
9. Amenorrhea (38 percent of celiacs vs. 9.2 percent of controls)
10. Anemia, folic acid deficiency, and iron deficiency, (along with elevated liver enzymes, one of the two most common laboratory abnormalities observed

in celiac disease; 6 percent of premenopausal women with anemias of unknown cause biopsy-proven celiac disease)

11. Anorexia nervosa/atypical eating disorders

12. Aphthous stomatitis/canker sores (up to 25 percent of celiac patients may
    have a history of oral ulceration)

13. Arthropathies (26 percent of CD patients with arthritic symptoms;
    41 percent if still eating gluten vs. 7.5 percent of controls):
    a. Arthritis, undifferentiated
    b. Arthralgia
    c. Polyarthritis, seronegative
    d. Juvenile arthritis
    e. Rheumatoid arthritis

14. Asperger's syndrome

15. Asthma

16. Ataxia

17. Atopic disorders:
    a. Allergic rhinitis
    b. Asthma
    c. Eczema
    d. Chronic urticaria

18. Attention deficit disorder (ADD)

19. Attention deficit hyperactivity disorder (ADHD)

20. Autism

21. Autoantibodies associated with celiac disease:
    a. IgA anti-gliadin antibodies
    b. IgG anti-gliadin antibodies
    c. IgA antiendomysium antibodies (autoantigen recently identified as the
       enzyme intestinal transglutaminase):
    d. IgA (and IgG) antireticulin antibodies
    e. Anti-transglutaminase IgA and IgG autoantibodies
    f. Anti-gastric inhibitory peptide (GIP) cell antibodies
    g. Anti-duodenal secretin cell autoantibodies
    h. Anti-enteroglucagon cell autoantibodies

    i. Anti-thyroid microsomal autoantibodies

    j. Anti-thyroid peroxidase autoantibodies (27 percent positive)

    k. Anti-gastric parietal cell autoantibodies

    l. Anti-adrenal cortex (suprarenal) autoantibodies

    m. Anti-pancreatic islet cell autoantibodies

    n. Anti-cardiolipin (14 percent of all CD patients)

    o. Anti-single-stranded DNA (14 percent of all CD patients)

    p. Anti-double-stranded DNA autoantibodies (23 percent)

    q. Anti-mitochondrial antibodies

    r. Cardiac-specific autoantibodies (in some cases of idiopathic dilated cardiomyopathy—see below)

    s. IgG anti-cell adhesion molecule desmoglein 3 in pemphigus vulgaris

22. Autoimmune diseases:

    a. Insulin-dependent diabetes mellitus (10 percent of all celiacs develop IDDM, up to 8 percent of IDDM patients have or will develop celiac disease; many authorities are now recommending that all IDDM patients be screened for CD annually for several years after IDDM diagnosis)

    b. Hyperthyroidism (3.7 percent of all celiacs) and hypothyroidism (8 percent of all celiacs); some authorities are now recommending that all autoimmune thyroid patients be routinely screened for celiac disease)

    c. Hypoparathyroidism

    d. Inflammatory bowel disorders

    e. Idiopathic Addison's disease

    f. Alopecia areata

    g. Vitiligo

    h. Systemic lupus erythematosus (SLE)

    i. Celiac disease (CD)

    j. Chronic active hepatitis

    k. Biliary cirrhosis, primary

    l. Dermatomyositis

    m. Pemphigus vulgaris (oral, esophageal, and anal lesions)

n. Myasthenia gravis

o. Autoimmune polyendocrine syndrome:

1. Hashimoto's thyroiditis with IDDM

2. Dermatitis herpetiformis with IDDM

p. Sjögren-Larsson syndrome

q. IgA nephropathy (Berger's disease)

23. Axonal neuropathy

24. Berger's disease/IgA nephropathy (Berger's is 6 times more frequent in males—5 percent of all primary glomerular diseases in United States, 10 to 20 percent in Europe, 30 to 40 percent in Asia)

25. Biliary cirrhosis, primary (autoimmune disease with antimitochondrial antibodies; primarily disease of women)

26. Biliary duct atresia (30 percent incidence in childhood CD)

27. Bone diseases:

a. Osteoporosis/lowered bone density in kids and adults

b. Osteopenia

c. Osteomalacia

d. Bone pain, "growing pains" in children

e. Bone fractures, pathological (from osteomalacia)

f. Elevated bone alkaline phosphatase

g. Hyperparathyroidism, secondary

h. Hypoparathyroidism, magnesium-deficiency induced

i. Elevated serum osteocalcin

j. Elevated urinary hydroxyproline excretion

k. Hypocalcemia

l. Hypocalcuria

28. Breast-feeding, absence of (up to 80 percent of CD children are not breast-fed, 96 percent breast-fed for 2 months or less)

29. Bullous pemphigoid

30. Calcium deficiency

31. Cancers:

a. Adenocarcinoma of small intestine

b. B-cell lymphoma

c. Bladder cancer

    d. Brain cancer

    e. Prostate cancer

    f. Squamous cell carcinoma of pharynx and esophagus

    g. T-cell lymphoma of small intestine (31 to 100 times more frequently found in celiac patients; new cases of non-Hodgkin's lymphoma are increasing by a little over .5 percent per year and deaths by 1.8 percent per year)

    h. Testicular cancer

32. Cardiomyopathy, idiopathic dilated (in children, 25 percent mortality rate the first year after diagnosis)

33. Celiac disease (CD):

    a. Classical active CD (gluten gastroenteropathy)

    b. Silent CD/subclinical gluten intolerance (typical CD mucosal histology with no abdominal symptoms)

    c. Latent CD (normal mucosa with positive serology initially; villous atrophy, mucosal crypt hyperplasia, intraepithelial lymphocyte infiltration develop later)

    d. Abortive type CD (transient/non-permanent—development of gluten tolerance later on)

    e. Potential CD

    f. CD in first-degree relatives (4.5 to 8.5 percent overall, 13.8 percent of siblings, 12 percent of offspring of celiacs, 70 percent of identical twins)

34. Cerebellar atrophy/cerebellar syndrome

35. Cerebral atrophy (central, cortical, and/or cerebellar)

36. Cerebral calcification (mostly occipital region)

37. Cerebral syndromes:

    a. Epilepsy

    b. Cerebral calcification

    c. Headache

    d. Mental deterioration

    e. Visual disturbances

38. Chest pain, noncardiac (see Esophageal symptoms)

39. Cholangitis, primary sclerosing

40. Cholecystokinin (CCK) inhibition (reduced CCK release from duode-

num with subsequent reduction in gallbladder emptying and pancreatic secretions)

41. Cirrhosis, primary biliary

42. Colitis, microscopic (27 percent with villous atrophy, 17 percent with CD-related serology, most with HLA-DQ genetic marker)

43. Crohn's disease

44. Cutaneous vasculitis

45. Dementia, intellectual impairment

46. Dental enamel lesions, permanent teeth (96 percent of CD children and 83 percent of CD adults with celiac-type color and structural defects, horizontal grooves, and/or vertical pits on one or more permanent teeth)

47. Depressive illness ("Depression is the most common symptom of gluten intolerance")

48. Dermatitis herpetiformis (classical non-GI manifestation of celiac disease; 25 percent without villous atrophy or crypt hyperplasia; instead only minor mucosal changes seen)

49. Diabetes mellitus, insulin-dependent (2.6 to 7.8 percent of IDDM children have CD—including silent and latent CD, 10 to 100 times higher prevalence of CD than expected)

50. Diarrhea, chronic

51. Down syndrome (prevalence of CD detected is 1 in 14)

52. Duodenal ulcers (antibiotic resistant)

53. Dysarthria

54. Dyslexia

55. Dysphagia (45 to 50 percent of CD patients—see Esophageal symptoms; when associated with iron deficiency, is called the Paterson-Brown Kelly [Plummer-Vinson] syndrome)

56. Eczema

57. Edema (in the more ill CD patients)

58. EEG abnormalities (may persist for 1 year on gluten-free diet)

59. Emotional and behavioral disorders:
    a. Irritability
    b. Querulousness, petulance
    c. Impulsivity

d. Depression (common presenting symptom of CD)

e. Anxiety

f. Aggressiveness

g. Autism

h. ADHD

i. Schizophrenia

60. Epilepsy:

a. Epilepsy associated with cerebral calcifications

b. Epilepsy associated with migraine headaches

c. Epilepsy associated with hyperactivity

d. Epilepsy associated with myoclonic ataxia (Ramsay Hunt's syndrome)

61. Esophageal symptoms (dysphagia, dysmotility, reflux esophagitis, heartburn, noncardiac chest pain)

62. Esophagitis, reflux (see Esophageal symptoms)

63. Eustachian tube dysfunction

64. Exorphin/opioidlike activity (gluten-induced)

65. Facial and hair features typical of CD:

a. Blue eyes and fair hair

b. Triangular-shaped face with prominent forehead and narrow jaw

c. Premature graying

66. Failure to thrive

67. Family members of celiac patients (parents and siblings)

68. Fatigue, chronic

69. Flatulence

70. Folic acid deficiency

71. Food sensitivities (soy, milk, monosodium glutamate, e.g.)

72. Gallbladder malfunction (impaired emptying, poor bile delivery, gallstones, e.g.)

73. Gastric inhibitory polypeptide reduction (inhibition of gut hormone release from upper small intestine)

74. Gastric ulcers

75. Gastrointestinal bleeding, occult (X-ray negative)

76. Gastrointestinal disorders:

a. Abdominal pain (up to 25 percent of CD patients complain of pain)

   b. Irritable bowel syndrome

   c. Crohn's disease

   d. Ulcerative colitis

   e. Chronic diarrhea

   f. Steatorhea

   g. Recurrent aphthous ulcers (canker sores)

   h. Nausea and vomiting

   i. Bloating, abdominal distension

   j. Flatulence

   k. GI bleeding

   l. Angular stomatitis

   m. Macroglossia

   n. Gastric ulcers

   o. Abnormal intestinal permeability (leaky gut)

   p. Pancreatic insufficiency

   q. Gut hormone inhibition (secretin, CCK, e.g.)

   r. Dyspepsia, esophageal reflux (5 percent of all such patients with gluten-induced duodenal villous atrophy)

77. Gastrointestinal polypeptide inhibition:

   a. Cholecystokinin

   b. Gastric inhibitory polypeptide

   c. Secretin

78. Genetics (see Human leukocyte antigens [HLA] below)

79. Glomerulonephritis, IgA-mediated

80. Grave's disease

81. Gynecological disorders:

   a. Amenorrhea

   b. Delayed menarche

   c. Delayed puberty

   d. Early menopause

82. Hair abnormalities:

   a. Alopecia areata

   b. Premature graying

83. Headaches (persistent, recurring, migrainelike, often not responsive to conventional therapies)
84. Heartburn (see Esophageal symptoms)
85. Heart disease:
    a. Ischemic heart disease, lower incidence of death in CD
    b. Cardiomyopathy, idiopathic dilated
    c. Chest pain, noncardiac (see Esophageal symptoms)
    d. Pericarditis, recurrent
86. Hematuria (macroscopic or microscopic)
87. Hepatitis, chronic active
88. Hepatitis, nonspecific reactive
89. Hormonal/endocrine abnormalities:
    a. Elevated plasma testosterone
    b. Reduced plasma dihydrotestosterone
    c. Elevated luteinizing hormone
    d. Hyperprolactinemia (associated with lowered CNS dopamine levels, a marker for active CD)
    e. Hyper- or hypoparathyroidism (associated with bone disease)
    f. Hypo- or hyperthyroidism
    g. Growth hormone deficiency
    h. Reduced secretin gut hormone blood levels
90. Human leukocyte antigens: HLA-DR3, DQ2, and B8 positive haplotypes (frequency of HLA-DR3 antigens in patients with CD is about 88 percent; normal population only 44 percent); HLA-DR3 and especially DQ2 antigens in diseases are thought to be associated with celiac disease:
    a. Celiac disease
    b. Dermatitis herpetiformis
    c. Multiple sclerosis
    d. Down syndrome
    e. Insulin-dependent diabetes mellitus (DR3 and B8 present in 86 percent of patients with both CD and IDDM; IDDM alone, 41 percent)
    f. Grave's disease
    g. Idiopathic Addison's disease

    h. Sicca syndrome

    i. Systemic lupus erythematosus

    j. Idiopathic IgA membranous nephropathy

    k. Myasthenia gravis

91. Hypertransaminasemia, alanine and aspartate (9 percent of all cases of hypertransaminasemia of unknown origin; found in about 50 percent of all celiac patients still on a gluten-containing diet; often found in otherwise symptom-free celiacs; returns to normal on gluten-free diet)

92. Hypoalbuminemia (in untreated celiac disease; returns to normal with a gluten-free diet)

93. Hypocalcemia

94. Hypocomplementemia

95. Hypogonadism

96. Hypoperfusion, frontal cortex of brain

97. Hyposplenism (10 percent of CD adults; remits on gluten-free diet)

98. IgA deficiency, total serum (3 percent frequency in both CD and IDDM vs. approximately 0.2 percent in normal population)

99. IgA nephropathy (see Nephropathies)

100. IgG and/or IgA anti-gliadin antibodies elevation (serum)

101. Impotence/loss of libido (19 percent of CD males are impotent)

102. Infertility in both women and men (2.1 million U.S. married couples are infertile—one-third male, one-third female, one-third both; 18 percent of all celiac males are infertile; abnormal sperm is reversed; a 50 percent increase in conception rate occurs on strict gluten-free diet)

103. Intellectual impairment/mental deterioration

104. Intraepithelial gamma/delta T-lymphocytes (increased density in mucosal epithelium)

105. Iron deficiency anemia (of unknown origin—very common in celiac patients)

106. Irritable bowel syndrome (IBS)

107. Ischemic heart disease (lower rate of death in CD patients)

108. Kidney disease (see Nephropathies)

109. Lactose intolerance (found in 50 percent of celiac patients)

110. Leaky gut syndrome/abnormal intestinal permeability
111. Lipofuscin storage (increased deposition in nerves, skin, and muscles)
112. Liver disease (15 times more frequent in CD; 47 percent of CD adults and 57 percent of CD children have evidence of liver impairment; biopsy-proven liver damage has been reported in most untreated CD patients):
    a. Abnormal function tests (elevated transaminases common extra-intestinal sign of CD)
    b. Biliary cirrhosis
    c. Chronic active hepatitis
    d. Nonspecific reactive hepatitis
113. Lupus erythematosus (0.3 to 1.3 percent of all CD patients)
114. Lymphocyte reactivity (reduced against tumors in CD)
115. Lymphocytic colitis (authorities recommend routine screening for CD)
116. Lymphocytic gastritis
117. Lymphomas (31 to 100 times more common in CD patients; risk returns to near normal with five years on a gluten-free diet)
118. Macroglossia (enlargement of the tongue)
119. Magnesium deficiency
120. Malabsorption:
    a. Low hemoglobin
    b. Reduced mean corpuscular volume (MCV)
    c. Low vitamin B_{12}
    d. Low folic acid
    e. Chronic diarrhea, flatulence
    f. Weight loss with wasting
    g. Chronic fatigue
121. Malabsorption syndrome (chronic diarrhea, flatulence, weight loss, and fatigue)
122. Malignancies (see both entries: Cancers and Lymphomas)
123. Malnutrition (deficiencies in iron, zinc, calcium, magnesium, potassium, and vitamins B_6, B_{12}, folic acid, A, D, E and/or K)
124. Mast cell degranulation
125. Menarche, delayed (delayed by over 1 year)

126. Menopause, early (occurs 2–4 years earlier in CD patients)
127. Mental symptoms and disorders:
     a. Inability to concentrate
     b. Mental deterioration
     c. Mental lethargy
     d. Distractibility
     e. Intelligence deficits
     f. Dementia
     g. Down syndrome
     h. ADHD
     i. ADD
     j. Autism
     k. Schizophrenia
128. Mesangial IgA deposits (often associated with celiac disease, Crohn's disease, adenocarcinomas, dermatitis herpetiformis, psoriasis, or IgA nephropathy)
129. Microscopic colitis (see Colitis)
130. Mineral deficiencies:
     a. Iron deficiency
     b. Calcium deficiency (hypocalcemia)
     c. Zinc deficiency
     d. Magnesium deficiency (hypomagnesemia)
     e. Potassium deficiency (hypokalemia)
     f. Selenium deficiency
131. Miscarriages
132. Mortality (a 1.9- to 3.4-fold increased mortality overall in adults—but not children, asymptomatic relatives, or those diagnosed by serology; death occurs most frequently within first to third year following diagnosis and then declines over time; highest death rates between ages 45–54 for men and 55–64 for women; major reported cause is intestinal lymphoma):
     a. A 31- to 100-fold increased risk of death from small intestinal lymphomas
     b. An 8.5-fold increased risk of death from esophageal cancer

    c. A 2.3-fold increased risk of death from all other malignant disease in CD men

    d. Chronic liver disease

    e. Lower death rate from ischemic heart disease and strokes than normal population

133. Multiple sclerosis

134. Myasthenia gravis

135. Mycosis fungoides

136. Myoclonic ataxia, progressive

137. Natural killer cell (reduced count)

138. Nephropathies:

    a. IgA nephropathy (Berger's disease)

    b. IgA glomerulonephritis

    c. Nephrotic syndrome

    d. Proteinuria

139. Neurological conditions, chronic, of unknown cause:

    a. Ataxia/myoclonic ataxia

    b. Axonal neuropathy

    c. Brain atrophy

    d. Cerebellar atrophy/cerebellar syndrome

    e. Epilepsy

    f. Hypoperfusion, frontal cortex

    g. Intellectual deterioration

    h. Multiple sclerosis

    i. Optic neuropathy

    j. Paresthesia

    k. Peripheral neuropathy

    l. Polyneuropathy

    m. Progressive neuromyopathy

    n. Ramsay Hunt's syndrome (epilepsy with myoclonic ataxia)

140. Obstetrical disorders:

    a. Recurrent abortions

    b. Stillbirths

    c. Infertility

    d. Subfertility

    e. Reduced time span of fertility

    f. Reduced pregnancy rate

141. Ocular myopathy

142. Opioidlike activity

143. Optic neuropathy

144. Osteocalcin elevation (serum)

145. Osteomalacia

146. Osteoporosis/osteopenia (70 percent of untreated CD patients with low bone density; in patients unresponsive to standard therapies—estrogen, vitamin D, calcium, bisphosphonates, calcitonin; bone density increases by 7.7 percent in 1 year on strict gluten-free diet alone)

147. Otitis media

148. Palmoplantar pustulosis (skin condition of soles and palms)

149. Pancreaticobiliary diseases:

    a. Pancreatic insufficiency

    b. Pancreatitis

    c. Papillary stenosis

    d. Papillitis

    e. Chronic duodenitis

    f. Impaired cholecystokinin release

150. Paresthesia

151. Pericarditis, recurrent

152. Pervasive developmental disorder

153. Polyarthritis, seronegative

154. Polymyositis

155. Polyneuropathy

156. Presenile dementia

157. Prolactin, elevated

158. Proteinuria (see Nephropathies)

159. Psoriasis

160. Psychiatric symptoms:

    a. Depression (common presenting symptom in celiac patients)

    b. Anxiety

161. Puberty, delayed

162. Ramsay Hunt's syndrome (epilepsy with myoclonic ataxia)

163. Rheumatoid arthritis (see Arthropathies)

164. Sarcoidosis (1.8 percent of all CD patients)

165. Secretin release inhibition (a 9-fold difference between untreated celiac and non-celiac following intraduodenal stimulation with HCl)

166. Secretory IgA deficiency (2.6 percent of CD patients are IgA deficient, 10 to 16 times higher than general population)

167. Selenium deficiency

168. Sexual behavior disorders (in untreated CD):

    a. Decreased frequency of sexual intercourse

    b. Decreased satisfaction from sexual intercourse

169. Short stature/growth failure (bone and growth retardation in children; celiac disease is a more common factor here than primary growth hormone deficiency)

170. Sicca syndrome

171. Sjögren-Larsson syndrome (2.9 percent of all CD patients and 15 percent of all Sjögren's patients with biopsy-proven celiac disease)

172. Skin diseases:

    a. Bullous pemphigoid

    b. Chronic urticaria

    c. Cutaneous vasculitis

    d. Dermatitis herpetiformis

    e. Eczema

    f. Psoriasis

    g. Palmoplantar pustulosis

173. Sperm abnormalities (reversed on gluten-free diet):

    a. Oligospermia (reduced sperm count)

    b. Abnormal sperm motility

    c. Abnormal sperm morphology

174. Steatorrhea

175. Stillbirths

176. Suicide

177. Thrombocytopenic purpura

178. Thyroid disease, autoimmune (up to 13 percent of all CDs; subclinical thyroid disease may be reversed in some cases within 1 year on gluten-free diet):

    a. Hypothyroidism (found in 5.8 to 8 perent of all celiac patients)

    b. Hyperthyroidism (found in 3.7 to 5 percent)

179. Turner's syndrome (a chromosomal disease associated with autoimmune disorders including thyroid disease, inflammatory bowel disease, diabetes, and juvenile rheumatoid arthritis; all overrepresented in celiac disease)

180. Ulcerative colitis

181. Urticaria (hives)

182. Vasculitis

183. Villous atrophy (partial/subtotal and total)

184. Vitamin deficiencies:

    a. Vitamin A deficiency

    b. Vitamin B_6 deficiency

    c. Vitamin B_{12} deficiency

    d. Folic acid deficiency

    e. Vitamin D deficiency

    f. Vitamin E deficiency

    g. Vitamin K deficiency (associated with nosebleeds, easy bruisability, internal hemorrhaging, and bone loss)

185. Vitiligo

186. Weight loss/failure to gain weight

187. Zinc deficiency

Heroic Thinkers and
Dietary Biases

Several heroic thinkers and researchers have blazed the trail past our cultural biases and preconceived notions. Their thoughtful observations and insightful interpretations of the health implications of gluten have opened the path to new insights that may help avert an epidemic in the offing for the twenty-first century. The stories of these courageous individuals have helped shape tomorrow's world of medicine. If we look at the evidence objectively, we can learn from them today.

STANISLAS TANCHOU (1791–1850)
Stanislas Tanchou was a visionary French physician who campaigned with Napoleon at Waterloo, then settled in Paris to practice medicine and do research. He conducted what may be the first detailed statistical study of the incidence of cancer deaths. He accumulated and analyzed data detailing the causes of death for people in Paris and surrounding rural areas over a period of eleven years. He also examined information about cancer found in ancient Egyptian mummies, along with

information that was then current from Egypt and Algiers. Tanchou's published findings over 150 years ago offer the first published evidence that implies that foods from grains contribute to cancer.

Tanchou offered the prophetic observation that "cancer is like insanity, found most often in the most civilized countries . . ."

VILHJALMUR STEFANSSON (1879–1962)

Another early researcher, an anthropology instructor at Harvard University named Vilhjalmur Stefansson, was one of the few to pay attention to Tanchou's ideas. His research, observations, deductions, and references regarding cancer are what led us to Tanchou's work. Stefansson left his teaching position in 1906 and traveled to the north coast of Canada to live among the Eskimos. He lived and worked among the Inuit, immersed in their way of life, for eleven of the twelve years between 1906 and 1918. Stefansson looked for but found no sign of cancer in the Stone-Age culture of the Inuit. He was the first to report on the healthfulness of this high-fat, high–animal protein diet in 1913. We would add that it was what the Inuits were not eating that also protected them from cancer; namely, the absence of gluten cereals.

Stefansson was also there to record the devastating loss of that protection, following adoption of a Western diet by these genetically ill-prepared northern natives. His observations, subsequent investigations, and their synthesis resulted in a theory of cancer that may hold the answer, even a cure, for many cancer patients. His theory is summarized in the title of his book, *Cancer: Disease of Civilization?*, and stands unchallenged. Cancer is a genetically influenced environmental disease of civilization.

SAMUEL GEE AND R. A. GIBBONS

In 1888, Dr. Samuel Gee provided a highly regarded, detailed description of classical celiac disease. One of Gee's contemporaries, R. A. Gibbons, believed this disease to be rare, afflicting only children. According to Gibbons, patients either recovered from this disease of childhood or they died. In either case, there would be little reason to look for it in adults.

Sadly, Gibbons's *very* narrow perspective and Gee's focus on the most dramatic cases resulted in perspectives that were to dominate medical thinking for more than a century. Even today, many U.S. practitioners still consider only childhood celiac disease to be a serious malady.

WHEAT-CELIAC CONNECTION AND WILLEM KAREL DICKE (1905–1962)

One of the greatest visionaries of the twentieth century was Dr. W. K. Dicke. His courageous pursuit of the underlying cause of celiac disease was a giant step toward recognition of the real nature of this disease. He invested much of his professional career to the solution of the celiac puzzle.

Dicke first began to suspect wheat as the cause of celiac disease when the mother of one patient suggested that possibility in 1932. Dicke stated: "As one frequently comes across the unfavorable influence of these nutrients, the conviction gradually grew within me that the observation mentioned above [that wheat might be the cause of celiac disease] was not any chance occurrence peculiar to a certain individual, but had something to do with the presence of celiac disease."

It is particularly interesting that Dicke says, when talking about bread, biscuits, and starches, that they are frequently seen as having an unfavorable influence. This original insight led to the monumental discovery that gluten is requisite to the manifestation of celiac disease.

Although there is some debate as to when Dr. Dicke first realized that wheat caused celiac symptoms, the evidence clearly indicates that he had done so by 1936. In keeping with a disgraceful tradition of attacking and abusing original thinkers going back countless centuries, Dr. Dicke was mocked and ridiculed when he tried to present his findings at a 1950 conference of gastroenterologists in New York City.

It was not until it became possible to confirm Dicke's findings through intestinal biopsies that his discovery began the agonizingly slow process of being accepted as the treatment of choice for celiac disease. The wheat-celiac connection, despite compelling evidence in support of it, continued to be a matter of debate in medical literature until 1964.

Unfortunately, some elements of the debate have continued outside the literature. There are dermatologists today who continue to treat the skin manifestation of celiac disease, called dermatitis herpetiformis, by prescribing steroid medications and/or dapsone instead of recommending a gluten-free diet. These drugs usually control the most obvious symptoms of this condition but do not address the cause. The dermatologists using this approach argue that it is unusual for patients to comply with a gluten-free diet, so the medication makes more sense. We, of course, vehemently disagree with this position, pointing to the increased risk of many cancers and autoimmune diseases and the protective benefits offered by a gluten-free diet.

SCHIZOPHRENIA CONNECTION AND
F. CURTIS DOHAN (1908–1991)

Medical science took yet another leap forward when Dr. F. Curtis Dohan learned that schizophrenia is frequently found in people with celiac disease, and celiac disease is frequently found in people with schizophrenia. Dohan was a prominent medical teacher, internist, and researcher who worked most of his illustrious forty-year career in the Philadelphia area. He has more than eighty publications in scientific journals to his credit. Dohan also enjoyed reading mystery stories, an interest that would ultimately benefit humanity. He found the association between schizophrenia and celiac disease intriguing. He pursued this medical puzzle with the same joy and interest that he used to solve the who-done-its in his leisure reading. His dogged pursuit of the schizophrenia-celiac connection is the wellspring of a whole new understanding of diet-induced mental illness, and his work serves as a model for investigating other dietary ailments.

In 1969, Dohan and his colleagues conducted an experiment. They reported significant improvements in hospitalized schizophrenic patients following a gluten-free and dairy-free diet. This report generated quite a lot of skepticism, but the results were soon repeated by M. Singh and S. Kay. The Dohan group's findings were repeated. Dohan subsequently conducted investigations showing that when gluten-containing grains are rare, schizophrenia is also rare.

In 1979, the discovery of morphinelike substances in partly digested gluten proteins, called gliadorphins or gluteomorphins, supported Dohan's work from a completely different direction. These morphinelike substances have been shown to interfere with the immune system, impact on blood vessel dilation, and alter chemical activity in the brain, thus acting as contributing factors in many psychiatric and brain illnesses, including learning and attention disorders, major depression, sleep disorders, postpartum psychosis, and autism.

AUTISM CONNECTION, PAUL SHATTOCK, AND KALLE REICHELT

Dr. Paul Shattock was a plant biochemist and lecturer at the University of Sunderland when his son was diagnosed with autism in 1974. He began collecting data on autism research. Then, Shattock heard speculation that autism is the result of peptide poisoning, following on Dohan's work. He began investigating the possibility that gluten and dairy were at the root of his son's ailment, and he has contributed important research that supports this hypothesis.

Dr. Kalle Reichelt, a researcher at the Pediatric Research Institute in Oslo, Norway, was also investigating peptides from gluten and dairy products in autistic patients. By 1990, Reichelt and Shattock had discovered that 90 percent of the autistic patients they studied had abnormally high levels of urinary peptides that they surmised were from dairy and gluten cereals.

These men, and now many other researchers, have established a connection between gluten consumption and several types of mental illness, behavioral problems, and learning disabilities. Broader recognition of these discoveries is slow. Given adequate time, we are confident that this work will become universally accepted. However, many concerned parents and others will want to act more quickly on this information, as the appropriate diet is very safe and nutritious. There is no downside to this therapy other than the inconvenience of implementing it while ensuring optimal nutrition. Those who currently suffer from these conditions will be unlikely to benefit from this information if they await its general acceptance before changing their diet.

NON-GLUTEN AGENTS OF DISEASE AND LOREN CORDAIN

Recent research conducted by Loren Cordain is also making headway in a broader area of gluten research. Cordain, a researcher at Colorado State University, has taken a more global approach to the evaluation of the impact of consuming gluten-containing grains. He has reported several antinutrients, psychoactive substances, and other non-gluten agents discovered in cereals, all of which can damage the human intestinal wall.

Cordain has also presented information about how we have made dramatic changes to the human diet since beginning cultivation of cereal grains ten thousand years ago and how those changes are now threatening to overwhelm us with chronic disease. Cordain has also debunked several myths regarding the diets of hunter-gatherers, showing that they were likely much more dependent on animal protein and fats than was previously believed.

All of these pioneering scientists, along with others too numerous to mention, have expanded human knowledge in this arena. Because of their diligence and considerable courage to think originally in the face of rejection and mockery, humanity is now offered an important choice.

The twentieth century's development of widespread consumption of highly processed foods brought with it a dramatic increase in gluten consumption. Examine the "ingredients" label on almost any processed food so you may see for yourself. Gluten and/or its derivatives are usually present. The view that these foods are healthy or at least not harmful helps to maintain many of the traditional forms of gluten consumption. Together, these and other factors have created the unprecedented level of gluten gluttony with which the industrial world entered the twenty-first century.

SOURCES

INTRODUCTION

Davidson, A. G., et al. "Screening for celiac disease." *Can Med Assoc J.* 1997; 157(5): 547–48.

Dicke, W. Coeliac disease: Investigation of the harmful effects of certain types of cereal on patients with coeliac disease, Ph.D. thesis, University of Utrecht. 1950.

Dickey, W., and Bodkin, S. "Prospective study of body mass index in patients with coeliac disease." *BMJ.* 1998 Nov 7; 317(7168): 1290.

Fasano, A. "Where have all the American celiacs gone?" *Acta Paediatr Suppl.* 1996 May; 412: 20–4.

Fine, K. D., Do, K., Schulte, K., Ogunji, F., Guerra, R., Osowski, L., and McCormack, J. "High prevalence of celiac sprue-like HLA-DQ genes and enteropathy in patients with the microscopic colitis syndrome." *Am J Gastroenterol.* 2000 Aug; 95(8): 1974–82.

Gibbons, R. "The coeliac affection in children." *Edinburgh Medical Journal* 1889; xxxv(iv): 321–30.

Hadjivassiliou, M., Grunewald, R. A., Davies-Jones, G. A. "Gluten sensitivity: A many-headed hydra." *BMJ.* 1999 Jun 26; 318(7200): 1710–11.

Marsh, M. N. "Gluten sensitivity and latency: Can patterns of intestinal antibody secretion define the great 'silent majority'?" *Gastroenterology.* 1993 May; 104(5): 1550–53.

Reading, C., and Meillon, R. *Your Family Tree Connection.* New Canaan, Conn.: Keats, 1988.

Selye, H. *Stress without Distress.* Philadelphia: Lippincott, 1974.

CHAPTER ONE

Allan, C., and Lutz, W. *Life Without Bread.* Chicago: Keats, 2000, p. 3.

Cordain, L. "Cereal grains: Humanity's double-edged sword." *World Rev Nutr Diet.* Simopopulos A. (ed.). 1999, vol. 84; Karger, Basel: 5, 6, 12, 13.

Diamond, J. *Guns, Germs, and Steel: The Fates of Human Societies.* New York: Norton & Co., 1997.

Eaton, S., and Konner, M. "Paleolithic nutrition." *NEJM.* 1985; 312(5): 283–89.

Eaton, S., and Nelson, D. "Calcium in evolutionary perspective." *Am J Clin Nutr.* 1991; 54: 281S–87S.

Egorov, T. A., Odintsova, T. I., and Musolyamov, A. K. "Determination of disulfide bonds in *gamma*-46 gliadin." *Biochemistry* (Mosc) 1999 Mar; 64(3): 294–7.

Erasmus, Udo. *Fats that Heal, Fats that Kill.* Vancouver, Canada: Alive Books, 1993.

Falchuk, Z. M., Katz, A. J., Shwachman, H., Rogentine, G. N., and Strober, W. "Gluten-sensitive enteropathy: Genetic analysis and organ culture study in 35 families." *Scand J Gastroenterol.* 1978; 13(7): 839–43.

Fine, K. D., Do, K., Schulte, K., Ogunji, F., Guerra, R., Osowski, L., and McCormack, J. "High prevalence of celiac sprue-like HLA-DQ genes and enteropathy in patients with the microscopic colitis syndrome." *Am J Gastroenterol.* 2000 Aug; 95(8): 1974–82.

Fukudome, S., and Yoshikawa, M. "Opioid peptides derived from wheat gluten: Their isolation and characterization." *Febs Letts.* 1992 Jan 13; 296(1): 107–11.

Harris, M. *Cannibals & Kings.* New York: Random House, 1977.

Hoggan, R. Application of the exorphin hypothesis to attention deficit disorder: A theoretical framework. M.A. thesis, University of Calgary, GDER, Calgary, Canada, 1998.

Kemppainen, T., Kroger, H., Janatuinen, E., Arnala, I., Kosma, V. M., Pikkarainen, P., Julkunen, R., Jurvelin, J., Alhava, E., and Uusitupa, M. "Osteoporosis in adult patients with celiac disease." *Bone.* 1999 Mar; 24(3): 249–55.

Larsen, C. S. Post-Pleistocene Human Evolution: Bioarchaeology of the Agricultural Transition. Fourteenth International Congress of Anthropological and Ethnological Sciences, Williamsburg, Virginia. 1998 July 26–Aug 1.

Leaky, R. *The Origin of Humankind.* New York: Basic Books, 1994.

Lewin, R. "A revolution of ideas in agricultural origins." *Science* 1988; 240: 984–86.

Lutz, W. "The colonization of Europe and our western diseases." *Medical Hypoth.* 1995; 45, 115–20.

Marsh, M. N. "Gluten sensitivity and latency. The histological background. Common food intolerances 1: Epidemiology of coeliac disease." *DYN Nutr Res.* 1992; vol. 2: 142–50.

Mora, S., et al. "Bone density and bone metabolism are normal after long-term gluten-free diet in young celiac patients." *Am J Gastroenterol.* 1999 Feb; 94(2): 398–403.

Mullis, K. *Dancing Naked in the Mindfield.* New York: Random House, 2000.

Neel, J. V. "When some fine old genes meet a 'new' environment." Simopopoulos AP (ed): Evolutionary aspects of nutrition and health, diet, exercise, genetics and chronic disease. *World Rev Nutr Diet.* 1999; Karger. Basel. 84: 1–18.

Rath, M., and Pauling, L. "Immunological evidence for the accumulation of lipoprotein (a) in the atherosclerotic lesion of the hypoascorbemic guinea pig." *Proc Natl Acad Sci USA.* 1990 Dec; 87(23): 9388–90.

Reeds, P. J. "Dispensable and indispensable amino acids for humans." *J Nutr.* 2000 Jul; 130(7): 1835S–40S. A review.

Richards, M., Corte-Real, H., Forster, P., Macaulay, V., Wilkinson-Herbots, H., Demaine, A., Papiha, S., Hedges, R., Bandelt, H. J., and Sykes, B. "Paleolithic and neolithic lineages in the European mitochondrial gene pool." *Am J Hum Genet.* 1996 Jul; 59(1): 185–203.

Shah, V. H., et al. "All that scallops is not celiac disease." *Gastrointest Endosc.* 2000 Jun; 51(6): 717–20.

Simoons, F. "Celiac disease as a geographic problem." In Walcher & Kretchmer (ed.). *Food Nutrition & Evolution.* New York: Masson, 1981.

Smith, J. M. *Shaping Life Genes, Embryos and Evolution.* London: Orion Publishing, 1998.

Stanford, C. *The Hunting Apes.* Princeton: Princeton University Press, 1999.

Stefansson, V. *Cancer: Disease of Civilization.* New York: Hill & Wang, 1960.

Stuart-Macadam, P. "Porotic hyperostosis: A new perspective." *Am J Phys Anthropol.* 1992 Jan; 87(1): 39–47.

Tortora, G., and Grabowski, S. *Principles of Anatomy and Physiology.* New York: HarperCollins, 1996, p. 704.

Ulijaszek, S. J. "Human dietary change." *Philos Trans R Soc Lond B Biol Sci.* 1991 Nov 29; 334(1270): 271–8 (with discussion on 278–9).

Williamson, D. *Celiac Disease: A Brief Overview in Celiac Disease Methods and Protocols.* M. N. Marsh (ed). Totowa, N.J.: Humana Press, 2000.

Zioudrou, C., Streaty, R. A., and Klee, W. A. "Opioid peptides derived from food proteins: The exorphins." *J Biol Chem.* 1979 Apr 10; 254(7): 2446–9.

CHAPTER 2

Anderson, C. "The evolution of a successful treatment for coeliac disease. Coeliac Disease." Marsh M. (ed.). *Blackwell Scientific.* London. 1992: 1–16.

British Museum. Dept. of Egyptian Antiquities: An introduction to ancient Egypt. London, 1979: 26–30.

Brothwell, D. *The Bio-cultural Background to Disease. Diseases in Antiquity.* Brothwell & Sandison (ed.). Springfield, Ill.: Thomas, 1967, 56–68.

Cooke, W., and Holmes, G. *Coeliac Disease.* Livingstone, N.Y.: Churchill, 1984, 1.

Cordain, L. "Cereal grains: Humanity's double-edged sword." *World Rev Nutr Diet.* A. Simopopulos (ed.). 1999, vol. 84; Karger, Basel: 5, 6, 12, 13.

Dicke, W. K. Coeliac disease: Investigation of the harmful effects of certain types of cereal on patients suffering from coeliac disease. Ph.D. thesis. in Medicine at University of Utrecht. 1950, C. J. Mulder (trans.), June 1, 1993.

Dohan, F. An internist looks at schizophrenia. Medical Affairs. University of Pennsylvania, Summer, 1972; 163.

Dohan, F., Grasberger, J., Lowell, F., Johnston, H., and Arbegast, A. "Relapsed schizophrenics: More rapid improvement on a milk- and cereal-free diet." *Brit J Psychiat.* 1969; 115: 595–96.

Dohan, F., Harper, E., Clark, M., Rodrigue, R., and Ziagas, V. "Is schizophrenia rare if grain is rare?" *Biol Psychiatry.* 1984; 19(3): 385–99.

Donadoni Roveri, A. *Egyptian Civilization.* Milan: Electa, 1987–1989; 20.

Eades, M. *Protein Power.* New York: Bantam Books, 1997.

Erasmus, U. *Fats that Heal, Fats that Kill.* Vancouver, Canada: Alive Books, 1996.

Gibbons, R. "The coeliac affection in children." *Edinburgh Medical Journal.* Oct 1889; XXXV(IV): 321–30.

Holmes, G., Prior, P., Lane, M., et al. "Malignancy in coeliac disease—effect of a gluten free diet." *Gut.* 1989; 30: 333–38.

Johnson-Kelly, L. "The evolutionary history of celiac disease." *J Pediatr Gastroenterol Nutr.* 2000; 31(3): S10.

Landis, S., Murray, T., Bolden, S., and Wingo, P. "Cancer statistics 1999." *CA Cancer J Clin.* 1999; 49(8): 8–31.

McCrone, J. "Gut Reaction." *New Scientist.* 1998 June 20: 42–45.

Moodey, R. L. *Roentgenologic Studies of Egyptian and Peruvian Mummies.* Chicago: Field Museum of Natural History, 1931.

Mycroft, F., Bernardin, J., and Kasarda, D. "MIF-like sequences in milk and wheat proteins." *NEJM.* 1982 Sep 30; 307(14): 895.

Papp, K. P. Dermatitis Herpetiformis. Canadian Celiac Association National Conference. Kitchener, Ontario. May 30, 1998.

Reichelt, K. personal communication.

Rowling, J. *Urology in Egypt: Diseases in Antiquity.* Brothwell & Sandison (ed.) Springfield, Ill.: Thomas, 1967, 494–97.

Ruffin, J., Carter, D., Johnston, D., and Baylin, G. "Gluten-free diet for nontropical sprue." *JAMA.* 1964 Apr 6: 162–64.

Sandison, A. *Degenerative Vascular Diseases in Antiquity.* Brothwell & Sandison (ed.). Springfield, Ill.: Thomas 1967, 478.

Sandison, A., and Wells, C. *Diseases of the Reproductive System.* Brothwell & Sandison (ed.). Springfield, Ill.: Thomas, 1967, 507.

Singh, M., and Kay, S. "Wheat gluten as a pathogenic factor in schizophrenia." *Science.* 1976; 191: 401–2.

Stefansson, V. *Cancer: Disease of Civilization?* New York: Hill & Wang, 1960, 26.

Swinson, C., Coles, E., Slavin, G., and Booth, C. "Coeliac disease and malignancy." *Lancet.* 1983; 1(8316): 111–15.

Tanchou, S. "Statistics of cancer." *Lancet* 1843 Aug 5: 593–94.

Van Berge-Henegouwen, CJJ Mulder. "Pioneer in the gluten free diet: Willem-Karel Dicke 1905–1962, over 50 years of gluten-free diet." *Gut.* 1993; 34: 1473–75.

Ventura, A., Magazzu, G., and Greco, L. "Duration of exposure to gluten and risk for autoimmune disorders in patients with celiac disease." *Gastroenterology.* 1999; 117: 297–303.

Wallace, A. "Dr. F. Curtis Dohan, Medical Researcher." *Philadelphia Inquirer.* Thursday, November 14, 1991.

Zioudrou, C., Streaty, R., and Klee, W. "Opioid peptides derived from food proteins." *J Biol Chem.* 1979; 254: 2446.

CHAPTER THREE

Auricchio, S., et al. "Gluten-sensitive enteropathy in childhood." *Pediatr Clin North Am.* 1988 Feb: 157–87.

Cacciari, E., et al. "Short stature and celiac disease: A relationship to consider even in patients with no gastrointestinal tract symptoms." *J Pediatr.* 1983 Nov: 708–11.

Collin, P., Hallstrom, O., Maki, M., Viander, M., and Keyrilainen, O. "Atypical coeliac disease found with serologic screening." *Scand J Gastroenterol.* 1990 Mar; 25(3): 245–50.

Delco, F., El-Serag, H. B., and Sonnenberg, A. "Celiac sprue among U.S. military veterans: Associated disorders and clinical manifestations." *Dig Dis Sci.* 1999 May; 44(5): 966–72.

Eichler, I., et al. "Growth failure and insulin-like growth factor (IGF-I) in childhood celiac disease." *Klin Wochenschr.* 1991 Nov 15: 825–29.

Fine, Kenneth, M.D. Private communication. July 2000.

Groll, A., et al. "Short stature as the primary manifestation of coeliac disease." *Lancet,* 1980 Nov 22: 1097.

Marsh, M. N., and Crowe, P. T. "Morphology of the mucosal lesion in gluten sensitivity." *Baillieres Clin Gastroenterol.* 1995 Jun; 9(2): 273–93.

Reading, R., Watson, J. G., Platt, J. W., and Bird, A. G. "Pulmonary hemosiderosis and gluten." *Arch Dis Child.* 1987 May; 62(5): 513–5.

Robertson, D. A., Taylor, N., Sidhu, H., Britten, A., Smith, C. L., and Holdstock, G. "Pulmonary permeability in coeliac disease and inflammatory bowel disease." *Digestion.* 1989; 42(2): 98–103.

Rosenbach, Y., et al. "Short stature as the major manifestation of celiac disease in older children." *Clin Pediatr.* (Phila). 1986 Jan: 13–16.

Stenhammar, L., et al. "Coeliac disease in children of short stature without gastrointestinal symptoms." *Eur J Pediatr.* 1986 Aug: 185–86.

Stevens, F. M., Connolly, C. E., Murray, J. P., and McCarthy, C. F. "Lung cavities in patients with coeliac disease." *Digestion.* 1990; 46(2): 72–80.

Tarlo, S. M., Broder, I., Prokipchuk, E. J., Peress, L., and Mintz, S. "Association between celiac disease and lung disease." *Chest.* 1981 Dec; 80(6): 715–8.

Williams, A. J. "Coeliac disease and allergic manifestations." *Lancet.* 1987 Apr 4; 1(8536): 808.

CHAPTER FOUR

Dickey, W., Hughes, D., and McMillan, S. "Reliance upon serum endomysial antibody testing underestimates the true prevalence of coeliac disease by one fifth." *Scand J Gastroenterol.* 2000; 35: 181–83.

Egan, C. A., Smith, E. P., Taylor, T. B., Meyer, L. J., Samowitz, W. S., and Zone, J. J. "Linear IgA bullous dermatosis responsive to a gluten-free diet." *Am J Gastroenterol.* 2001 Jun; 96(6): 1927–9.

Loft, D. E., Marsh, M. N., Sandle, G. I., Crowe, P. T., Garner, V., Gordon, D., and Baker, R. "Studies of intestinal lymphoid tissue. XII. Epithelial lymphocyte and mucosal responses to rectal gluten challenge in celiac sprue." *Gastroenterology.* 1989 Jul; 97(1): 29–37.

Marsh, M. N. "Gluten, major histocompatibility complex, and the small intestine. A molecular and immunobiologic approach to the spectrum of gluten sensitivity ('celiac sprue')." *Gastroenterology.* 1992 Jan; 102(1): 330–54.

Mulder, C. J. J., Rostami, K., and Marsh, M. N. "When is a coeliac a coeliac?" *Gut.* April 1998; 42: 594.

Seissler, J., Boms, S., Wohlrab, U., Morgenthaler, N. G., Mothes, T., Boehm, B. O., and Scherbaum, W. A. "Antibodies to human recombinant tissue transglutaminase measured by radioligand assay: Evidence for high diagnostic sensitivity for celiac disease." *Horm Metab Res.* 1999 Jun; 31(6): 375–9.

Chapter Five

Chartrand, L. J., Russo, P. A., Duhaime, A. G., and Seidman, E. G. "Wheat starch intolerance in patients with celiac disease." *J Am Diet Assoc.* 1997 Jun; 97(6): 612–8.

Kaukinen, K., Collin, P., Holm, K., Rantala, I., Vuolteenaho, N., Reunala, T., and Maki, M. "Wheat starch-containing gluten-free flour products in the treatment of coeliac disease and dermatitis herpetiformis. A long-term follow-up study." *Scand J Gastroenterol.* 1999 Feb; 34(2): 163–9.

Musselman, B. C., Wenzel, J. E., and Groover, R. V. "Potassium-depletion paralysis associated with gluten-induced enteropathy." *Am J Dis Child.* 1968: 116; 414–17.

Chapter Six

Addolorato, G., Stefanini, G. F., Capristo, E., Caputo, F., Gasbarrini, A., and Gasbarrini, G. "Anxiety and depression in adult untreated celiac subjects and in patients affected by inflammatory bowel disease: A personality 'trait' or a reactive illness?" *Hepatogastroenterology.* 1996 Nov–Dec; 43(12): 1513–7.

Altuntas, B., Filik, B., Ensari, A., Zorlu, P., and Tezic, T. "Can zinc deficiency be used as a marker for the diagnosis of celiac disease in Turkish children with short stature?" *Pediatr Int.* 2000 Dec; 42(6): 682–84.

Alwitry, A. "Vitamin A deficiency in coeliac disease." *Brit J Ophthalmol.* 2000 Sep; 84(9): 1079–80.

Annibale, B., Severi, C., Chistolini, A., Antonelli, G., Lahner, E., Marcheggiano, A., Iannoni, C., Monarca, B., and Fave, G. D. "Efficacy of gluten-free diet alone on recovery from iron deficiency anemia in adult celiac patients." *Am J Gastroenterol.* 2001 Jan; 96(1): 132–7.

Bakalkin, G., Demuth, H., and Nyberg, F. "Relationship between primary structure and activity in exorphins and endogenous opioid peptides." *Febs Letts.* 1992; 310(1): 13–16.

Beck, S. A., and Tisdale, M. J. "Effect of insulin on weight loss and tumour growth in a cachexia model." *Br J Cancer.* 1989 May; 59(5): 677–81.

Black, Paul. "Psychoneuroimmunology: Brain and immunity." *Sci Am*. 1995; 2(6): 16–25.

Boda, M., and Nemeth, I. "Decrease in the antioxidant capacity of red blood cells in children with celiac disease." *Acta Paediatr Hung*. 1992; 32(3): 241–55.

Briggs, J., McKerron, C., Souhami, R., Taylor, D., and Andrews, H. "Severe systemic infections complicating 'mainline' heroin addiction." *Lancet*. 1967 Dec 9: 1227–8.

Brown, S., Stimmel, B., Taub, R., Kochwa, S., and Rosenfield, R. "Immunologic dysfunction in heroin addicts." *Arch Intern Med*. 1974; 134: 1001–6.

Carter, K., and Carter, B. *Childbed Fever: A Scientific Biography of Ignaz Semmelweis*. Westport, Conn.: Greenwood Press, 1994.

Castany, M. A., Nguyen, H. H., Pospisil, M., Fric, P., and Tlaskalova-Hogenova, H. "Natural killer cell activity in coeliac disease: Effect of in vitro treatment on effector lymphocytes and/or target lymphoblastoid, myeloid and epithelial cell lines with gliadin." *Folia Microbiol (Praha)*. 1995, 40(6): 615–20.

Chang, K., Su, Y., Brent, D., and Chang, J. "Isolation of a specific u-Opiate receptor peptide, morphiceptin, from an enzymatic digest of milk proteins." *J Biol Chem*. 1985; 260(17): 9706–12.

Cohen, M. *Health and the Rise of Civilization*. New Haven, Conn.: Yale University Press, 1989, 109.

Colquhoun, I., and Bunday, S. "A lack of essential fatty acids as a possible cause of hyperactivity in children." *Med Hypotl*. 1981; 7: 673–9.

Cooke, W., and Holmes, G. *Coeliac Disease*. Livingstone, N.Y.: Churchill, 1984, 248.

Cuoco, L., Cammarota, G., Tursi, A., Papa, M., Certo, R., Cianci, G., Fedeli, G., and Gasbarrini, G. "Disappearance of gastric mucosa-associated lymphoid tissue in coeliac patients after gluten withdrawal." *Scand J Gastroenterol*. 1998; 33(4): 401–5.

Dahele, A., and Ghosh, S. "Vitamin B12 deficiency in untreated celiac disease." *Am J Gastroenterol*. 2001 Mar; 96(3): 745–50.

de Boer, W., Maas, M., and Tytgat, G. "Disappearance of mesenteric lymphadenopathy with gluten-free diet in celiac sprue." *J Clin Gastroenterol*. 1993; 16 (4): 317–9.

De Santis, A., Addolorato, G., Romito, A., Caputo, S., Giordano, A., Gambassi, G., Taranto, C., Manna, R., and Gasbarrini, G. "Schizophrenic symptoms and SPECT abnormalities in a coeliac patient: Regression after a gluten-free diet." *J Intern Med.* 1997 Nov; 242(5): 421–3.

Di Sabatino, A., Bertrandi, E., Casadei Maldini, M., Pennese, F., Proietti, F., and Corzza, G. R. "Phenotyping of periperal blood lymphocytes in adult coeliac disease." *Immunology.* 1998; 95(4): 572–6.

Dickey, W., and Bodkin, S. "Prospective study of body mass index in patients with coeliac disease." *BMJ.* 1998 Nov 7; 317(7168): 1290.

Dohan, C. "Genetic hypothesis of idiopathic schizophrenia: Its exorphin connection." *Schiz Bull.* 1988; 14(4): 489–94.

Dohan, F. C. "Genetics and idiopathic schizophrenia." *Am J Psych.* 1989; 146(11): 1522–3.

Dohan, F. C. "Is celiac disease a clue to the pathogenesis of schizophrenia?" *Mental Hyg.* 1969 Oct; 53(4): 525–9.

Donahoe, R. M., Falek, A., Madden, J. J., Nicholson, J. K., Bokos, P., Gallegos, K., and Veit, R. "Effects of cocaine and other drugs of abuse on immune function." *Adv Exp Med Biol.* 1991; 288: 143–50.

Donaldson, S. S. "Effect of nutrition as related to radiation and chemotherapy." *Nutrition and Cancer,* Winick (ed.). New York: Wiley & Sons, 1977, 137–53.

Duesberg, P. *Inventing the AIDS Virus.* Washington, D.C.: Regnery, 1995, 424.

Dwyer, J. T. "Nutrition support of HIV+ patients." *Henry Ford Hosp Med J.* 1991; 39(1): 60–5.

Eaton, B., and Konner, M. "Paleolithic nutrition." *NEJM.* 1985; 312(5): 283–9.

Edwards, C., Williams, A., and Asquith, P. "Bronchopulmonary disease in coeliac patients." *J Clin Pathol.* 1985 Apr; 38(4): 361–7.

Egan, L., Stevens, F., and McCarthy, C. "Celiac disease and T cell lymphoma." *NEJM.* 1996; 335(21).

Eisenstein, T., and Hilburger, M. "Opioid modulation of immune responses: Effects on phagocyte and lymphoid cell populations." *J Neuroimmunol.* 1998; 83(1–2): 36–44.

Falek, A., Donahoe, R. M., Madden, J. J., and Shafer, D. A. "Opiates as immuno-suppressive and genotoxic agents." *Adv Exp Med Biol.* 1991; 288: 189–201.

Fasano, A., Not, T., Wang, W., Uzzau, S., Berti, I., Tommasini, A., and Goldblum, S. E. "Zonulin, a newly discovered modulator of intestinal permeability and its expression in coeliac disease." *Lancet.* 2000 Apr 29; 355(9214): 1518–9.

Fine, Kenneth, M.D. Private communication. July 2000.

Freier, D., and Fuchs, B. "A mechanism of action for morphine-induced immuno-suppression: Corticosterone mediates morphine-induced suppression of natural killer cell activity." *JPET.* 1994; 270: 1127–33.

Fukudome, S., Jinsmaa, Y., Matsukawa, T., Sasaki, R., and Yoshikawa, M. "Release of opioid peptides, gluten exorphins by the action of pancreatic elastase." *Febs Letts.* 1997; 412: 475–9.

Fukudome, S., Shimatsu, A., Suganuma, H., and Yoshikawa, M. "Effect of gluten exorphins A5 and B5 on the post prandial plasma insulin level in conscious rats." *Life Sci.* 1995; 57(7): 729–34.

Fukudome, S., and Yoshikawa, M. "Gluten exorphin C. A novel opioid peptide derived from wheat gluten." *Febs Lets.* 1993 Jan 18; 316(1): 17–9.

Fukudome, S., and Yoshikawa, M. "Opioid peptides derived from wheat gluten. Their isolation and characterization." *Febs Letts.* 1992; 296(1): 107–11.

Fundia, A., Gomez, J. C., Maurino, E., Boerr, L., Bai, J. C., Larripa, I., and Slavutsky, I. "Chromosome instability in untreated adult celiac disease patients." *Acta Paediatr Suppl.* 1996 May; 412: 82–4.

Fundia, A. F., Gonzalez Cid MB, Bai, J., Gomez. J. C., Mazure, R., Vazquez, H., Larripa, I. B., and Slavutsky, I. R. "Chromosome instability in lymphocytes from patients with celiac disease." *Clin Genet.* 1994 Feb; 45(2): 57–61.

Geller, S., and Stimmel, B. "Diagnostic confusion from lymphatic lesions in heroin." *Ann Int Med.* 1973, 78: 703–5.

Govitrapong, P., Suttitum, T., Kotchabhakdi, N., and Uneklabh, T. "Alterations of immune functions in heroin addicts and heroin withdrawal subjects." *J Pharmacol Exp Ther.* 1998 Aug; 286(2): 883–9.

Harper, D., Nisbet, R., and Siegert, R. "Dietary gluten and learning to attend to redundant stimuli." *Biol Psychiatry.* 1997; 42: 1060–6.

Harris, P., and Ferguson, L. "Dietary fibres may protect or enhance carcinogenesis." *Mutat Res.* 1999 July 15; 443(1–2): 95–110.

Harris, P., and Garret, R. "Susceptibility of addicts to infection and neoplasia." *NEJM.* 1972; 287(6): 310.

"Hemoptysis, pulmonary infiltrates, and diarrhea in a 36-year-old man." *Am J Med.* 1986 May; 80(5): 930–8.

Hoggan, R. "Absolutism's hidden message for medical scientism." *Interchange.* 1997; 28(2–3): 18–19.

Hoggan, R. "Considering wheat, rye, and barley proteins as aids to carcinogens." *Med Hypoth.* 1997 Sep; 49(3): 285–8.

Holmes, G., Prior, P., Lane, M., et al. "Malignancy in coeliac disease—effect of a gluten free diet." *Gut.* 1989; 30: 333–8.

Holmes, G. K. "Celiac disease and malignancy." *J Pediatr Gastroenterol Nutr.* 1997 May; 24(5): S20–3.

Horvath, K., Graf, L., Walcz, E., Bodanszky, H., and Schuler, D. "Naloxone antagonizes effect of alpha-gliadin on leucocyte migration in patients with coeliac disease." *Lancet.* 1985 Jul 27; 2(8448): 184–5.

Huebner, F., Lieberman, K. W., Rubino, R. P., and Wall, J. S. "Demonstration of high opioid-like activity in isolated peptides from wheat gluten hydrolysates." *Peptides.* 1984 Nov–Dec; 5(6): 1139–47.

Jain, M., Hislop, G., Howe, G., and Ghadirian, P. "Plant foods, antioxidants, and prostate cancer risk: Findings from case-control studies in Canada." *Nutr Cancer.* 1999; 34(2): 173–84.

Jameson, S. "Coeliac disease, insulin-like growth factor, bone mineral density, and zinc." *Scand J Gastroenterol.* 2000 Aug; 35(8): 894–6.

Johnston, S. D., and Watson, R. G. "Small bowel lymphoma in unrecognized coeliac disease: A cause for concern?" *Eur J Gastroenterol Hepatol.* 2000 Jun; 12(6): 645–8.

Knivsberg, A. M. "Urine patterns, peptide levels and IgA/IgG antibodies to food proteins in children with dyslexia." *Pediatr Rehabil.* 1997 Jan–Mar; 1(1): 25–33.

Kozlowska, Z. E. "Evaluation of mental status of children with malabsorption syndrome after long-term treatment with gluten-free diet (preliminary report)." *Psychiatr Pol.* (Polish) 1991 Mar–Apr; 25(2): 130-4.

Kristensen, P., Andersen, A., and Irgens, L. "Hormone-dependent cancer and adverse reproductive outcomes in farmers' families—effects of climactic conditions favoring fungal growth in grain." *Scand J Work Environ. Health* 2000; 26(4): 331–7.

Layon, J., Idris, A., Warzynski, M., Sherer, R., Brauner, D., Patch, O., McCulley, D., and Orris, P. "Altered T-lymphocyte subsets in hospitalized intravenous drug abusers." *Arch Intern Med.* 1984 Jul; 144(7): 1376–80.

Lodyga-Chruscinska, E., Micera, G., Szajdzinska-Pietek, E., and Sanna, D. "Copper(II) complexes of opiate-like food peptides." *J Agric Food Chem.* 1998; 46: 115–8.

Lopez, M. C., Huang, D. S., Watzl, B., Chen, G. J., and Watson, R. R. "Splenocyte subsets in normal and protein malnourished mice after long-term exposure to cocaine or morphine." *Life Sci.* 1991; 49(17): 1253–62.

Loukas, S., Varoucha, D., Zioudrou, C., Streaty, R., and Klee, A. "Opioid activities and structures of a-casein-derived exorphins." *Biochemistry.* 1983; 22: 4567–73.

Louria, D., Hensle, T., and Rose, J. "The major medical complications of heroin addiction." *Ann Int Med.* 1967; 67(1): 1–22.

Maclaurin, B., Cooke, W., and Ling, N. "Impaired lymphocyte reactivity against tumour cells in patients with coeliac disease." *Gut.* 1971; 12: 794–800.

Madden, J. J., Falek, A., Donahoe, R., Ketelson, D., and Chappel, C. L. "Opiate binding sites on cells of the immune system." *NIDA Res Monogr.* 1991; 105: 103–8.

McDonough, R. J., Madden, J. J., Falek, A., Shafer, D. A., Pline, M., Gordon, D., Bokos, P., Kuehnle, J. C., and Mendelson, J. "Alteration of T and null lymphocyte frequencies in the peripheral blood of human opiate addicts: In vivo evidence for opiate receptor sites on T lymphocytes." *J Immunol.* 1980 Dec; 125(6): 2539–43.

Meisel, H. "Chemical characterization and opioid activity of an exorphin isolated from in vivo digests of casein." *Febs Letts.* 1986; 196(2): 223–7.

Morley, J. "Food peptides." *JAMA.* 1982; 247(17): 2379–80.

Morley, J., Levine, A., Yamada, T., Gebhard, R., Prigge, W., Shafer, R., Goetz, F., and Silvis, S. "Effect of exorphins on gastrointestinal function, hormonal release and appetite." *Gastroenterology.* 1983; 84(6): 1517–23.

Munchau, A., and Vogel, P. "Reversible posterior encephalopathy possibly related to coeliac disease: A vitamin-depleted brain?" *Eur Neurol.* 9; 41(4): 232–4.

Murray, J. A. "The widening spectrum of celiac disease." *Am J Clin Nutr.* 1999 Mar; 69(3): 354–65.

Mycroft, F., Bernardin, J., and Kasarda, D. "MIF-lide sequences in milk and wheat proteins." *N Engl J Med.* 1982 Sep 30; 307(14): 895.

Mycroft, F. J., Bhargava, H. N., and Wei, E. T. "Pharmacological activities of the MIF-1 analogues Pro-Leu-Gly, Tyr-Pro-Leu-Gly and pareptide." *Peptides.* 1987 Nov–Dec; 8(6): 1051–5.

Nebeling, L. C., and Lerner, E. "Implementing a ketogenic diet based on medium-chain triglyceride oil in pediatric patients with cancer." *J Am Diet Assoc.* 1995 Jun; 95(6): 693–7.

Nebeling, L. C., Miraldi, F., Shurin, S. B., and Lerner, E. "Effects of a ketogenic diet on tumor metabolism and nutritional status in pediatric oncology patients: Two case reports." *J Am Coll Nutr.* 1995 Apr; 14(2): 202–8.

Nedvidkova, J., Kasafirek, E., Dlavac, A., and Felt, V. "Effect of beta-casomorphin and its analog on serum prolactin in the rat." *Exp Clin Endocrinol.* 1985; 85(2): 249–52.

Odetti, P., Valentini, S., Aragno, I., Garibaldi, S., Pronzato, M. A., Rolandi, E., and Barreca, T. "Oxidative stress in subjects affected by celiac disease." *Free Radical Res.* 1998 Jul; 29(1): 17–24.

Oikarinen, A., and Raitio, A. "Melanoma and other skin cancers in circumpolar areas." *Int J Circumpolar Health.* 2000 Jan; 59(1): 52–56.

Palacio, A., Tamariz, L., Berger, J., and Patarca, R. "Enteropathy-associated T-cell lymphoma and its immunocarcinogenic correlates: Case report and review of the literature." *Crit Rev Oncog.* 1998; 9(1): 63–81.

Pirozhkov, S. V., Watson, R. R., and Chen, G. J. "Ethanol enhances immunosuppression induced by cocaine." *Alcohol Suppl.* 1993; 2: 75–82.

Quesnel, A., Moja, P., Lucht, F., Touraine, J. L., Pozzetto, B., and Genin, C. "Is there IgA of gut mucosal origin in the serum of HIV1 infected patients?" *Gut.* 1994 Jun; 35(6): 803–8.

Quinones-Galvan, A., Lifshitz-Guinzberg, A., Ruiz-Arguelles, G. J. "Gluten-free diet for AIDS-associated enteropathy." *Ann Int Med.* 1990 Nov 15; 113(10): 806–7.

Reading, C., and Meillon, R. *Your Family Tree Connection.* New Canaan, Conn.: Keats, 1988.

Ricca, V., Mannucci, E., Calabro, A., Bernardo, M. D., Cabras, P. L., and Rotella, C. M. "Anorexia nervosa and celiac disease: Two case reports." *Int J Eat Disord.* 2000 Jan; 27(1): 119–22.

Roe, D. *A Plague of Corn: The Social History of Pellagra.* Ithaca, N.Y.: Cornell University Press, 1973.

Sabita, R., Ramakrishanan, S., Loh, H., and Lee, N. "Chronic morphine treatment selectively suppresses macrophage colony formation in bone marrow." *Eu J Pharmacol.* 1991; 195: 359–63.

Sailstad, D. M., Boykin, E. H., Slade, R., Doerfler, D. L., and Selgrade, M. K. "The effect of a vitamin A acetate diet on ultraviolet radiation-induced immune suppression as measured by contact hypersensitivity to mice." *Photolhem Photobiol.* 2000 Dec; 72(6): 766–71.

Schreinemachers, D. "Cancer mortality in four northern wheat-producing states." *Environmental Health Perspectives.* 2000; 108(9): 873–81.

Schusdziarra, V., Henrichs, I., Holland, A., Klier, M., and Pfeiffer, E. "Evidence for an effect of exorphins on plasma insulin and glucagon levels in dogs." *Diabetes.* 1981 30 April: 362–4.

Schusdziarra, V., Holland, A., Schick, R., de la Fuente, A., Klier, M., Naier, V., Brantl, V., and Pfeiffer, E. "Modulation of post-prandial insulin release by ingested opiate-like substances in dogs." *Diabotologia.* 1983; 24: 113–6.

Schusdziarra, V., Schick, R., de la Fuente, A., Holland, A., Brantl, V., and Pfeiffer, E. "Effect of beta-casomorphins on somatostatin release in dogs." *Endocrinology.* 1983; 112: 1948–51.

Scott, H., and Brandtzaeg, P. "Pathogenesis of food protein intolerance." *Acta Paediatr Scand Suppl.* 1989; 351: 48–52.

Selby, P. L., Davies, M., Adams, J. E., and Mawer, E. B. "Bone loss in celiac disease is related to secondary hyperparathyroidism." *J Bone Miner Res.* 1999 Apr; 14(4): 652–7.

Shafer, D. A., Falek, A., Donahoe, R. M., and Madden, J. J. "Biogenetic effects of opiates." *Int J Addict.* 1990; 91; 25(1A): 1–18.

Shavit, Y., Depaulis, A., Martin, F. C., Terman, G. W., Pechnick, R. N., Zane, C. J., Gale, R. P., and Liebeskind, J. C. "Involvement of brain opiate receptors in the immune-suppressive effect of morphine." *Proc Natl Acad Sci USA.* 1986 Sep; 83(18): 7114–7.

Simonati, A., Battistella, P. A., Guariso, G., Clementi, M., and Rizzuto, N. "Coeliac disease associated with peripheral neuropathy in a child: A case report." *Neuropediatrics.* 1998 Jun; 29(3): 155–8.

Slattery, M. L. "Diet, lifestyle, and colon cancer." *Semin Gastrointest Dis.* 2000 Jul; 11(3): 142–6.

Smith, W., Glauser, F., Dearden, L., Wells, I., Novey, H., McRae, D., Reid, J., and Newcomb, K. "Deposits of immunoglobulin and complement in the pulmonary tissue of patients with 'heroin lung'." *Chest.* 1978; 73(4): 471–6.

Smyth, P. P., Shering, S. G., Kilbane, M. T., Murray, M. J., McDermott, E. W., Smith, D. F., and O'Higgins, N. J. "Serum thyroid peroxidase autoantibodies, thyroid volume, and outcome in breast carcinoma." *J Clin Endocrinol Metab.* 1998 Aug; 83(8): 2711–6.

Sollid, L. M. "Molecular basis of celiac disease." *Ann Rev Immunol.* 2000; 18: 53–81.

Stazi, A. V., and Mantovani, A. "A risk factor for female fertility and pregnancy: Celiac disease." *Gynecol Endocrinol.* 2000 Dec; 14(6): 454–63.

Stevens, F. M., Connolly, C. E., Murray, J. P., and McCarthy, C. F. "Lung cavities in patients with coeliac disease." *Digestion.* 1990; 46(2): 72–80.

Stokes, P. L., Prior, P., Sorahan, T. M., McWalter, R. J., Waterhouse, J. A., and Cooke, W. T. "Malignancy (in relatives of patients with coeliac disease)." *Br J Prev Soc Med.* 1976 Mar; 30(1): 17–21.

Swinson, C., Coles, E., Slavin, G., and Booth, C. "Coeliac disease and malignancy." *Lancet.* 1983; 1(8316): 111–5.

Tanchou, S. "Statistics of Cancer." *Lancet.* 1843 Aug 5; 593.

Tigh, M., and Ciclitira, P. "The implications of recent advances in coeliac disease." *Acta Paediatr.* 1993; 82: 805–10.

Tisdale, M. J., and Brennan, R. A. "A comparison of long-chain triglycerides and medium-chain triglycerides on weight loss and tumour size in a cachexia model." *Br J Cancer.* 1988 Nov; 58(5): 580–3.

Tortora and Anagnostakos. *Principles of Anatomy and Physiology,* 6th ed. New York: Harper & Row, 1990, 674.

Toscano, V., Conti, F. G., Anastasi, E., Mariani, P., Tiberti, C., Poggi, M., Montuori, M., Monti, S., Laureti, S., Cipolletta, E., Gemme, G., Caiola, S., Di Mario, U., and Bonamico, M. "Importance of gluten in the induction of endocrine autoantibodies and organ dysfunction in adolescent celiac patients." *Am J Gastroenterol.* 2000 Jul; 95(7): 1742–8.

Vahidy, R., and Akbar, S. "Lymphocyte sub-populations in a group of heroin addicts in Pakistan." *Ann Acad Med Singapore.* 1990; 19(6): 823–6.

Vineis, P., Crosignani, P., Sacerdote, C., Fontana, A., Masala, G., Miligi, L., Nanni, O., Ramazzotti, V., Rodella, S., Stagnaro, E., Tumino, R., Vigano, C., Vindigni, C., and Costantini, A. S. "Haematopoietic cancer and medical history: A multicentre case control study." *J Epidemiol Community Health.* 2000 Jun; 54(6): 431–6.

Wadley, G., and Martin, A. "The origins of agriculture—a biological perspective and a new hypothesis." *Australian Biologist.* 1993; 6: 96–105.

Wood, N. C., Hamilton, I., Axon, A. T., Khan, S. A., Quirke, P., Mindham, R. H., McGuigan, K., and Prison, H. M. "Abnormal intestinal permeability: An etiological factor in chronic psychiatric disorders?" *Br J Psychiat.* 1987 Jun; 150: 853–6.

Wright, D., Jones, D., Clark, H., Mead, G., Hodges, E., and Howell, W. "Is adult-onset coeliac disease due to a low-grade lymphoma of intraepithelial T lymphocytes?" *Lancet.* 1991; 337(June 8): 1373–4.

Wright, D., Jones, D., and Mead, G. "Coeliac disease and lymphoma." *Lancet* 1991; 337: 1373.

Wright, D. "The major complications of coeliac disease." *Baillieres Clin Gastroenterol.* 1995 Jun; 9(2): 351–69.

Zioudrou, C., Streaty, R., and Klee, W. "Opioid peptides derived from food proteins. *J Biol. Chem.* 1979; 254: 2446–9.

CHAPTER SEVEN

Atkinson, M. A., and Eisenbarth, G. S. "Type 1 diabetes: New perspectives on disease pathogenesis and treatment." *Lancet.* 2001 Jul 21; 358(9277): 221–9.

Borg, A. A., Dawes, P. T., Swan, C. H., and Hothersall, T. E. "Persistent monoarthritis and occult coeliac disease." *Postgrad Med J.* 1994 Jan; 70(819): 51–53.

Bourne, Ann. Rheum Dis 1985; Bugnato Rheumatol Int 2000; *Slot Locht Scand J Rheumatol.* 2000; *Evron J Rheumatol.* 1996; Chakravarty & Scott br. *J Rheumatol.* 1992.

Collin, P., Salmi, J., Hallstrom, O., Reunala, T., and Pasternack, A. "Autoimmune thyroid disorders and coeliac disease." *Eur J Endocrinol.* 1994 Feb; 130(2): 137–40.

Cooke and Holmes. *Coeliac Disease.* Livingstone, N.Y.: Churchill, 1984.

Cordain, L., Toohey, L., Smith, M. J., and Hickey, M. S. "Modulation of immune function by dietary lectins in rheumatoid arthritis." *Br J Nutr.* 2000 Mar; 83(3): 207–17.

Cuoco, L., Certo, M., Jorizzo, R. A., DeVitis, I., Tursi, A., Papa, A., De Marinis, L., Fedeli, P., Fedeli, G., and Gasbarrini, G. "Prevalence and early diagnosis of coeliac disease in autoimmune thyroid disorders." *Ital J Gastroenterol Hepatol.* 1999 May; 31(4): 283–7.

Cuoco, L., Jorizzo, R. A., De Vitis, I., Cammarota, G., Fedeli, G., and Gasbarrini, G. "Celiac disease and autoimmune endocrine disorders." *Dig Dis Sci.* 2000 Jul; 45(7): 1470–1.

de Vos, R. J., de Boer, W. A., and Haas, F. D. "Is there a relationship between psoriasis and coeliac disease?" *J Intern Med.* 1995 Jan; 237(1): 118.

Falcini, F., Ferrari, R., Simonini, G., Calabri, G. B., Pazzaglia, A., and Lionetti, P. "Recurrent monoarthritis in an 11-year-old boy with occult coeliac disease. Successful and stable remission after gluten-free diet." *Clin Exp Rheumatol.* 1999 Jul–Aug; 17(4): 509–11.

Hagander, B., Berg, N. O., Brandt, L., Norden, A., Sjolund, K., and Stenstam, M. "Hepatic injury in adult coeliac disease." *Lancet.* 1977 Aug 6; 2(8032): 270–2.

Horvath, K., and Mehta, D. I. "Celiac disease—a worldwide problem." *Indian J Pediatr.* 2000 Oct; 67(10): 757–63.

Imramovska, M., Benes, Z., Krupickova, S., and Tlaskalova-Hogenova, H. "Occurrence of IgA and IgG autoantibodies to calreticulin in coeliac disease and various autoimmune diseases." *J Autoimmun.* 2000 Dec; 15(4): 441–9.

Kaukinen, K., Collin, P., Mykkanen, A. H., Partanen, J., Maki, M., and Salmi, J. "Celiac disease and autoimmune endocrinologic disorders." *Dig Dis Sci.* 1999 Jul; 44(7):1428–33.

Kjeldsen-Kragh, J., Haugen, M., Borchgrevink, C. F., Laerum, E., Eek, M., Mowinkel, P., Hovi, K., and Forre, O. "Controlled trial of fasting and one-year egetarian diet in rheumatoid arthritis." *Lancet.* 1991 Oct 12; 38(8772): 899–902.

Lepore, L., Martelossi, S., Pennesi, M., Falcini, F., Ermini, M. L., Ferrari, R., Perticarari, S., Presani, G., Lucchesi, A., Lapini, M., and Ventura, A. "Prevalence of celiac disease in patients with juvenile chronic arthritis." *J Pediatr.* 1996 Aug; 129(2): 311–3.

Lepore, L., Pennesi, M., Ventura, A., Torre, G., Falcini, F., Lucchesi, A., and Perticarari, S. "Anti-alpha-gliadin antibodies are not predictive of celiac disease in juvenile chronic arthritis." *Acta Paediatr.* 1993 Jun–Jul; 82(6–7): 569–73.

Lubrano, E., Ciacci, C., Ames, P. R., Mazzacca, G., Oriente, P., and Scarpa, R. "The arthritis of coeliac disease: Prevalence and pattern in 200 adult patients." *Br J Rheumatol.* 1996 Dec; 35(12): 1314–8.

Luzi, L., Perseghin, G., Brendel, M. D., Terruzzi, I., Battezzati, A., Eckhard, M., Brandhorst, D., Brandhorst, H., Friemann, S., Socci, C., Di Carlo, V., Piceni Sereni, L., Benedini, S., Secchi, A., Pozza, G., and Bretzel, R. G. "Metabolic effects of restoring partial beta-cell function after islet allotransplantation in type 1 diabetic patients." *Diabetes.* 2001 Feb; 50(2): 277–82.

Michaelsson, G., and Gerden, B. "How common is gluten intolerance among patients with psoriasis?" *Acta Derm Venereol.* 1991; 71(1): 90.

Michaelsson, G., Gerden, B., Hagforsen, E., Nilsson, B., Pihl-Lundin, I., Kraaz, W., Hjelmquist, G., and Loof, L. "Psoriasis patients with antibodies to gliadin can be improved by a gluten-free diet." *Br J Dermatol.* 2000 Jan; 142(1): 44–51.

Natter, S., Granditsch, G., Reichel, G. L., Baghestanian, M., Valent, P., Elfman, L., Gronlund, H., Kraft, D., and Valenta, R. "IgA cross-reactivity between a nuclear autoantigen and wheat proteins suggests molecular mimicry as a possible pathomechanism in celiac disease." *Eur J Immunol.* 2001 Mar; 31(3): 918–28.

O'Farrelly, C., Marten, D., Melcher, D., McDougall, B., Price, R., Goldstein, A. J., Sherwood. R., and Fernandes, L. "Association between villous atrophy in rheumatoid arthritis and a rheumatoid factor and gliadin-specific IgG." *Lancet.* 1988 Oct 8; 2(8615): 819–22.

O'Farrelly, C., Price, R., McGillivray, A. J., and Fernandes, L. "IgA rheumatoid factor and IgG dietary protein antibodies are associated in rheumatoid arthritis." *Immunol Invest.* 1989 Jul; 18(6): 753–64.

Paimela, L., Kurki, P., Leirisalo-Repo, M., and Piirainen, H. "Gliadin immune reactivity in patients with rheumatoid arthritis." *Clin Exp Rheumatol.* 1995 Sep–Oct; 13(5): 603–7.

Pellegrini, G., Scotta, M. S., Soardo, S., Avanzini, M. A., Ravelli, A., Burgio, G. R., and Martini, A. "Elevated IgA anti-gliadin antibodies in juvenile chronic arthritis." *Clin Exp Rheumatol.* 1991 Nov–Dec; 9(6): 653–6.

Sategna-Guidetti, C., Volta, U., Ciacci, C., Usai, P., Carlino, A., De Franceschi, L., Camera, A., Pelli, A., and Brossa, C. "Prevalence of thyroid disorders in untreated adult celiac disease patients and effect of gluten withdrawal: An Italian multicenter study." *Am J Gastroenterol.* 2001 Mar; 96(3): 751–7.

Scott, F. W. "Food-induced type 1 diabetes in the BB rat." *Diabetes Metab Rev.* 1996 Dec; 12(4): 341–59.

Scott, F. W., Cloutier, H. E., Kleemann, R., Woerz-Pagenstert, U., Rowsell, P., Modler, H. W., and Kolb, H. "Potential mechanisms by which certain foods promote or inhibit the development of spontaneous diabetes in BB rats: Dose, timing, early effect on islet area, and switch in infiltrate from Th1 to Th2 cells." *Diabetes.* 1997 Apr; 46(4): 589–98.

Sjöberg, K., Lindgren, S., and Eriksson, S. "Frequent occurrence of non-specific gliadin antibodies in chronic liver disease. Endomysial but not gliadin antibodies predict coeliac disease in patients with chronic liver disease." *Scand J Gastroenterol.* 1997 Nov; 32(11): 1162–7.

Toscano, V., Conti, F. G., Anastasi, E., Mariani, P., Tiberti, C., Poggi, M., Montuori, M., Monti, S., Laureti, S., Cipolletta, E., Gemme, G., Caiola, S., Di Mario, U., and Bonamico, M. "Importance of gluten in the induction of endocrine auto-antibodies and organ dysfunction in adolescent celiac patients." *Am J Gastroenterol.* 2000 Jul; 95(7): 1742–8.

Tuckova, L., Tlaskalova-Hogenova, H., Farre, M. A., Karska, K., Rossmann, P., Kolinska, J., and Kocna, P. "Molecular mimicry as a possible cause of autoimmune reactions in celiac disease? Antibodies to gliadin cross-react with epitopes on enterocytes." *Clin Immunol Immunopathol.* 1995 Feb; 74(2): 170–6.

Unsworth, D. J., and Walker-Smith, J. A. "Autoimmunity in diarrheal disease." *J Pediatr Gastroenterol Nutr.* 1985 Jun; 4(3): 375–80.

Vajro, P., Fontanella, A., Mayer, M., De Vincenzo, A., Terracciano, L. M., D'Armiento, M., and Vecchione, R. "Elevated serum aminotransferase activity as an early manifestation of gluten-sensitive enteropathy." *J Pediatr.* 1993 Mar; 122(3): 416–9.

Ventura, A., Magazzu, G., and Greco, L. "Duration of exposure to gluten and risk for autoimmune disorders in patients with celiac disease. SIGEP Study Group for Autoimmune Disorders in Celiac Disease." *Gastroenterology.* 1999 Aug; 117(2): 297–303.

Volta, U., De Franceschi, L., Lari, F., Molinaro, N., Zoli, M., and Bianchi, F. B. "Coeliac disease hidden by cryptogenic hypertransaminasaemia." *Lancet*. 1998 Jul 4; 352(9121): 26–29.

Volta, U., De Franceschi, L., Molinaro, N., Cassani, F., Muratori, L., Lenzi, M., Bianchi, F. B., and Czaja, A. J. "Frequency and significance of anti-gliadin and anti-endomysial antibodies in autoimmune hepatitis." *Dig Dis Sci*. 1998 Oct; 43(10): 2190–5.

Winer, S., Astsaturov, I., Cheung, R., Gunaratnam, L., Kubiak, V., Cortez, M. A., Moscarello, M., O'Connor, P. W., McKerlie, C., Becker, D. J., and Dosch, H. M. "Type I diabetes and multiple sclerosis patients target Islet plus central nervous system autoantigens; nonimmunized nonobese diabetic mice can develop autoimmune encephalitis." *J Immunol*. 2001 Feb 15; 166(4): 2831–41.

CHAPTER EIGHT

Corazza, G. R., Di Sario, A., Cecchetti, L., Tarozzi, C., Corrao, G., Bernardi, M., and Gasbarrini, G. "Bone mass and metabolism in patients with celiac disease." *Gastroenterology*. 1995 Jul; 109(1): 122–8.

Feskanich, D., Weber, P., Willett, W. C., Rockett, H., Booth, S. L., and Colditz, G. A. "Vitamin K intake and hip fractures in women: A prospective study." *Am J Clin Nutr*. 1999 Jan; 69(1): 74–79.

Kemppainen, T., Kroger, H., Janatuinen, E., Arnala, I., Lamberg-Allardt, C., Karkkainen, M., Kosma, V. M., Julkunen, R., Jurvelin, J., Alhava, E., and Uusitupa, M. "Bone recovery after a gluten-free diet: A 5-year follow-up study." *Bone*. 1999 Sep; 25(3): 355–60.

National Osteoporosis Foundation. http://www.nof.org/osteoporosis/stats.htm.

Wortsman, J., and Kumar, V. "Case report: Idiopathic hypoparathyroidism coexisting with celiac disease: Immunologic studies." *Am J Med Sci*. 1994 Jun; 307(6): 420–7.

CHAPTER NINE

Battistella, P. A., Mattesi, P., Casara, G. L., Carollo, C., Condini, A., Allegri, F., and Rigon, F. "Bilateral cerebral occipital calcifications and migraine-like headache." *Cephalalgia*. 1987 Jun; 7(2): 125–9.

Bostwick, H. E., Berezin, S. H., Halata, M. S., Jacobson, R., and Medow, M. S.

"Celiac disease presenting with microcephaly." *J Pediatr.* 2001 Apr; 138(4): 589–92.

Bye, A. M., Andermann, F., Robitaille, Y., Oliver, M., Bohane, T., and Andermann, E. "Cortical vascular abnormalities in the syndrome of celiac disease, epilepsy, bilateral occipital calcifications, and folate deficiency." *Ann Neurol.* 1993 Sep; 34(3): 399–403.

Cernibori, A., and Gobbi, G. "Partial seizures, cerebral calcifications and celiac disease." *Ital J Neurol Sci.* 1995 Apr; 16(3): 187–91.

Challacombe, D. N., and Wheeler, E. E. "Are the changes of mood in children with coeliac disease due to abnormal serotonin metabolism?" *Nutr Health.* 1987; 5(3–4): 145–52.

Collin, P., Pirttila, T., Nurmikko, T., Somer, H., Erila, T., and Keyrilainen, O. "Celiac disease, brain atrophy, and dementia." *Neurology.* 1991 Mar; 41(3): 372–5.

Colquhoun, I., and Bunday, S. "A lack of essential fatty acids as a possible cause of hyperactivity in children." *Med Hypoth.* 1981 May; 7(5): 673–9.

Corvaglia, L., Catamo, R., Pepe, G., Lazzari, R., and Corvaglia, E. "Depression in adult untreated celiac subjects: Diagnosis by the pediatrician." *Am J Gastroenterol.* 1999 Mar; 94(3): 839–43.

Cronin, C. C., Jackson, L. M., Feighery, C., Shanahan, F., Abuzakouk, M., Ryder, D. Q., Whelton, M., and Callaghan, N. "Coeliac disease and epilepsy." *QJM.* 1998 Apr; 91(4): 303–8.

De Santis, A., Addolorato, G., Romito, A., Caputo, S., Giordano, A., Gambassi, G., Taranto, C., Manna, R., and Gasbarrini, G. "Schizophrenic symptoms and SPECT abnormalities in a coeliac patient: Regression after a gluten-free diet." *J Intern Med.* 1997 Nov; 242(5): 421–3.

Dohan, F. "An internist looks at schizophrenia." *Medical Affairs.* 1972. University of Pennsylvania, 163, 7–11.

Dohan, F., Grassberger, J., Lowell, F., Johnson, H., and Arbegast, A. "Relapsed schizophrenics: More rapid improvement on a milk- and cereal-free diet." *Brit J Psych.* 1969; 115: 595–6.

Gibbons, R. "The Coeliac Affection in Children." *Edinburgh Medical Journal.* 1889; xxxv (iv): 321–30.

Gobbi, G., Bouquet, F., Greco, L., Lambertini, A., Tassinari, C. A., Ventura, A., and

Zaniboni, M. G. "Coeliac disease, epilepsy, and cerebral calcifications. The Italian working group on coeliac disease and epilepsy." *Lancet.* 1992 Aug 22; 340(8817): 439–43.

Grech, P., Richards, J., McLaren, S., and Winkelman, J. "Psychological sequelae and quality of life in coeliac disease." *J Pediatr Gastroenterol Nutr.* 2000; 31(Suppl. 3): S4.

Hadjivassiliou, M., Gibson, A., Davies-Jones, G. A., Lobo, A. J., Stephenson, T. J., and Milford-Ward, A. "Does cryptic gluten sensitivity play a part in neurological illness?" *Lancet.* 1996 Feb 10; 347(8998): 369–71.

Hadjivassiliou, M., Grunewald, R. A., and Davies-Jones, G. A. "Idiopathic cerebellar ataxia associated with celiac disease: Lack of distinctive neurological features." *J Neurol Neurosurg Psych.* 1999 Aug; 67(2): 257.

Hadjivassiliou, M., Grunewald, R. A., Lawden, M., Davies-Jones, G. A., Powell, T., and Smith, C. M. "Headache and CNS white matter abnormalities associated with gluten sensitivity." *Neurology.* 2001 Feb 13; 56(3): 385–8.

Hernandez, M. A., Colina, G., and Ortigosa, L. "Epilepsy, cerebral calcifications and clinical or subclinical coeliac disease. Course and follow-up with gluten-free diet." *Seizure.* 1998 Feb; 7(1): 49–54.

Holmes, G. K. "Non-malignant complications of coeliac disease." *Acta Paediatr Suppl.* 1996 May; 412: 68–75.

Horvath, K., Papadimitriou, J. C., Rabsztyn, A., Drachenberg, C., and Tildon, J. T. "Gastrointestinal abnormalities in children with autistic disorder." *J Pediatr.* 1999; 135: 559–63.

Knivsberg, A. M. "Urine patterns, peptide levels and IgA/IgG antibodies to food proteins in children with dyslexia." *Pediatr Rehabil.* 1997 Jan–Mar; 1(1): 25–33.

Kozlowska, Z. E. [Evaluation of mental status of children with malabsorption syndrome after long-term treatment with gluten-free diet (preliminary report)]. *Psychiatr Pol.* 1991 Mar–Apr; 25(2): 130–4.

Kristoferitsch, W., and Fointner, H. "Progressive cerebellar syndrome in adult coeliac disease." *J Neurol.* 1987 Feb; 234(2): 116–8.

La Mantia, L., Pollo, B., Savoiardo, M., Costa, A., Eoli, M., Allegranza, A., Boiardi, A., and Cestari, C. "Meningocortical calcifying angiomatosis and celiac disease." *Clin Neurol Neurosurg.* 1998 Sep; 100(3): 209–15.

Lea, M. E., Harbord, M., and Sage, M. R. "Bilateral occipital calcification associated with celiac disease, folate deficiency, and epilepsy." *AJNR Am J Neuroradiol.* 1995 Aug; 16(7): 1498–500.

Macdonald, C. E., and Playford, R. J. "Iron deficiency anaemia and febrile convulsions . . . and coeliac disease." *BMJ.* 1996 Nov 9; 313(7066): 1205.

MacDougall, R. "My Fight Against Multiple Sclerosis." Regencies, Inc., 1980.

Magaudda, A., Dalla Bernardina, B., De Marco, P., Sfaello, Z., Longo, M., Colamaria, V., Daniele, O., Tortorella, G., Tata, M. A., Di Perri, R., et al. "Bilateral occipital calcification, epilepsy and coeliac disease: Clinical and neuroimaging features of a new syndrome." *J Neurol Neurosurg Psych.* 1993 Aug; 56(8): 885–9.

Manikam, R. "Behavioral medicine approaches to celiac disease." *J Pediatr Gastroenterol Nutr.* 2000; 31(Suppl. 3): S9.

Marziani, E., and Pianaroli, A. "Celiac disease in a 3-year-old child: Psychological issues can often divert diagnosis." *J Pediatr Gastroenterol Nutr.* 2000; 31 (Suppl. 3): S14.

Matheson, N. A. "Letter: Multiple sclerosis and diet." *Lancet.* 1974 Oct 5; 2 (7884): 831.

Matthews-Larson, J. *Seven Weeks to Sobriety.* New York: Fawcett Columbine, 1992, 32–41.

Moss, G. *Mental Disorders in Antiquity, Diseases in Antiquity.* Brothwell & Sandison (eds). Springfield, Il.: Thomas, 1967; (55), 716.

Mustalahti, K., Lohiniemi, S., Collin, P., and Maki, M. "Improving quality of life of silent celiac disease (CD) patients during gluten-free diet warrants screening." *J Pediatr Gastroenterol Nutr.* 2000; 31(Suppl. 3): S7.

Paul, K., Todt, J., and Eysold, R. [EEG research findings in children with celiac disease according to dietary variations]. *Zeitschrift der Klinische Medizin.* 1985; 40: 707–9.

Pratesi, R., Gandolfi, L., Friedman, H., Farage, L., de Castro, C. A., and Catassi, C. "Serum IgA antibodies from patients with coeliac disease react strongly with human brain blood-vessel structures." *Scand J Gastroenterol.* 1998 Aug; 33(8): 817–21.

Reichelt, K. L., Hole, K., Hamberger, A., Saelid, G., Edminson, P. D., Braestrup, C. B., Lingjaerde, O., Ledaal, P., and Orbeck, H. "Biologically active peptide-containing fractions in schizophrenia and childhood autism." *Adv Biochem Psychopharmacol.* 1981; 28: 627–43.

Reichelt, K. L., and Stensrud, M. "Increase in urinary peptides prior to the diagnosis of schizophrenia." *Schizophr Res.* 1998 Nov 30; 34(3): 211–3.

Reichelt, K. L., and Teigland-Gjerstad, B. "Decreased urinary peptide excretion in schizophrenic patients after neuroleptic treatment." *Psychiatry Res.* 1995 Sep 29; 58(2): 171–6.

Revnova, M., and Homan, L. "Clinical aspects of coeliac disease (CD) in children in Russia." *J Pediatr Gastroenterol Nutr.* 2000; 31(Suppl. 3): S6.

Rostami, K., and Leyten, Q. "Epilepsy resulted from folic acid/vitamin B-12 deficiency caused by celiac disease." *J Pediatr Gastroenterol Nutr.* 2000; 31 (Supp 3): S6.

Singh, M., and Kay, S. "Wheat gluten as a pathogenic factor in schizophrenia." *Science.* 1976; 191: 401–2.

Thibault, L., Coulon, J., and Roberge, C. "Changes in serum amino acid content and dopamine-B-hydroxylase activity and brain neurotransmitter interaction in cats fed casein with or without gluten or gliadin." *J Clin Biochem Nutr.* 1988; 4: 209–221.

Trygstad, O. E., Reichelt, K. L., Foss, I., Edminson, P. D., Saelid, G., Bremer, J., Hole, K., Orbeckm II., Johansen, J. H., Boler, J. B., Titlestad, K., and Opstad, P. K. "Patterns of peptides and protein-associated-peptide complexes in psychiatric disorders." *Br J Psychiat.* 1980 Jan; 136: 59–72.

Wakefield, et al. "New variant of IBD observed in children with developmental disorders." *Am J Gastroenterol.* 2000; 95: 2154–6, 2285–95.

Yacyshyn, B., Meddings, J., Sadowski, D., and Bowen-Yacyshyn, M. B. "Multiple sclerosis patients have peripheral blood CD45RO+ B cells and increased intestinal permeability." *Dig Dis Sci.* 1996 Dec; 41(12): 2493–8.

CHAPTER TEN

"A 37-year-old woman with liver disease and recurrent diarrhea." *N Engl J Med.* 1999 Nov 11; 341(20): 1530–7.

Case records of the Massachusetts General Hospital. Weekly clinicopathological exercises. Case 34-1999.

Dohan, F., Grassberger, J., Lowell, F., Johnson, H., and Arbegast, A. "Relapsed schizophrenics: More rapid improvement on a milk- and cereal-free diet." *Brit J Psych.* 1969; 115: 595–6.

Fhahdazkhani, B., Maghari, M., Nasseri Moghaddam, S., Kamalin, N., Sotoudeh, M., Minapour, M., and Malekzadeh, R. "Prevalence of celiac disease among Iranian patients with chronic diarrhea." Abstract #3 *JPGN.* 2000 Sept; 31: S3–S29.

Fine, K. D., Do, K., Schulte, K., Ogunji, F., Guerra, R., Osowski, L., and McCormack, J. "High prevalence of celiac sprue-like HLA-DQ genes and enteropathy in patients with the microscopic colitis syndrome." *Am J Gastroenterol.* 2000 Aug; 95(8): 1974–82.

Koninckx, C. R., Giliams, J. P., Polanco, I., and Pena, A. S., "IgA antigliadin antibodies in celiac and inflammatory bowel disease." *J Pediatr Gastroenterol Nutr.* 1984 Nov; 3(5): 676–82.

Murray, J. Road to Wellness. National Conference of the Canadian Celiac Association. 1999 May.

Sanders, D., Carter, M., Dharan, M., Miford-Ward, A., McAlindon, M., and Lobo, A. "The prevalence of celiac disease in irritable bowel syndrome." Abstract #76 *JPGN.* 2000 Sept; 31: S3–S29.

Stenner, P. H., Dancey, C. P., and Watts, S. "The understanding of their illness amongst people with irritable bowel syndrome: A Q methodological study." *Soc Sci Med.* 2000 Aug; 51(3): 439–52.

Vahedi, H., Minapoor, M., and Malekzadeh, R. "Should IBS patients be screened for celiac disease?" Abstract #2 *JPGN.* 2000 Sept; 31: S3–S29.

CHAPTER ELEVEN

Ackerson and Resnick. "The effects of l-glutamine, n-acetyl-d-glucosamine, gamma-linoleic acid and gamma oryzanol on intestinal permeability." *Townsend Letter for Doctors.* 1993 January.

Belli et al. "Chronic intermittent elemental diet improves failure in children with Crohn's disease." *Gastroenterology.* 1988; vol. 94: 603–10.

Bodvarsson, S., Jonsdottir, I., Freysdottir, J., Leonard, J. N., Fry, L., and Valdimarsson, H. "Dermatitis herpetiformis—an autoimmune disease due to cross-reaction between dietary glutenin and dermal elastin?" *Scand J Immunol.* 1993 Dec; 38(6): 546–50.

Byrne et al. "Growth hormone, glutamine and fiber enhance adaptation of remnant bowel following massive intestinal resection." *Surg Forum 43*. 1992; 151–3.

De Blaauw, I., et al. "Glutamine depletion and increased gut permeability in non-anorectic, non-weight-losing tumor-bearing rats." *Gastroenterology*. 1997 January; 112(1): 118–26.

De Vincenzi, M., Luchetti, R., Peruffo, A. D., Curioni, A., Pogna, N. E., and Gasbarrini, G. "In vitro assessment of acetic-acid-soluble proteins (glutenin) toxicity in celiac disease." *J Biochem Toxicol*. 1996; 11(4): 205–10.

Elia, M., and Lunn, P. G. "The use of glutamine in the treatment of gastrointestinal disorders in man. *Nutrition*. 1997 Jul; 13(7–8): 743–7.

Furst, P., et al. "Glutamine dipeptides in clinical nutrition." *Nutrition*, 1997: 13 (7/8): 731–7.

Komatsu, S., and Hiranom H. "Rice seed globulin: A protein similar to wheat seed glutenin." *Phytochemistry*. 1992 Oct; 31(10): 3455–9

Li, I, et al. "Glutamine prevents parenteral nutrition-induced increases in intestinal permeability." *Journal of Parenteral and Enteral Nutrition*. 1994; 18: 3030–307.

MacBurney, M. B. A., et al. "A cost-evaluation of glutamine-supplemented parenteral nutrition in adult bone marrow transplant patients." *J Am Diet Assoc*. 1994 Nov; 94(11): 1263–6.

Messing, B., et al. "Whole-body protein metabolism assessed by leucine and glutamine kinetics in adult patients with active celiac disease." *Metabolism*. 1998 Dec, 47:12, 1429–33.

Neu, J. "Enteral glutamine supplementation for very low birth weight infants decreases morbidity." *J Pediatr*. 1997; 131: 691–9.

van de Wal, Y., Kooy, Y. M., van Veelen, P., Vader, W., August, S. A., Drijfhout, J. W., Pena, S. A., and Koning, F. "Glutenin is involved in the gluten-driven mucosal T cell response." *Eur J Immunol*. 1999 Oct; 29(10): 3133–9.

Van der Hulst, R. R. W. J. .et al. "Glutamine and intestinal immune cells in humans." *Journal of Parenteral and Enteral Nutrition*. 1997; 21(6): 310–5.

Windmueller, H. G., and Spaeth, A. E. "Identification of ketone bodies and glutamine as the major respiratory fuels in vivo for post-absorptive rat small intestine." *J Biol Chem*. 1978; 253: 69–76.

APPENDIX E

Anderson, C. "The evolution of a successful treatment for coeliac disease." Marsh M. (ed.). *Blackwell Scientific.* 1992: 1–16.

Dicke, W. K. Coeliac disease: Investigation of the harmful effects of certain types of cereal on patients suffering from coeliac disease. Ph.D. thesis in Medicine at University of Utrecht. 1950, transl. C. J. Mulder, June 1, 1993.

Dohan, F. An Internist looks at schizophrenia. Medical Affairs. University of Pennsylvania, Summer, 1972; 163.

Dohan, F., Grasberger, J., Lowell, F., Johnston, H., and Arbegast, A. "Relapsed schizophrenics: More rapid improvement on a milk- and cereal-free diet." *Brit J Psychiat.* 1969; 115: 595–6.

Dohan, F., Harper, E., Clark, M., Rodrigue, R., and Ziagas, V. "Is schizophrenia rare if grain is rare?" *Biol Psychiatry.* 1984; 19(3): 385–99.

Erasmus, U. *Fats that Heal, Fats that Kill.* Vancouver, Canada: Alive Books, 1996.

Gibbons, R. "The coeliac affection in children." *Edinburgh Medical Journal.* 1889 Oct; XXXV(IV): 321–30.

Holmes, G., Prior, P., Lane, M., et al. "Malignancy in coeliac disease—effect of a gluten free diet." *Gut.* 1989; 30: 333–8.

Landis, S., Murray, T., Bolden, S., and Wingo, P. "Cancer Statistics 1999." *CA Cancer J. Clin.* 1999; 49(8): 8–31.

Papp, K. P. Dermatitis Herpetiformis. Canadian Celiac Association National Conference. Kitchener, Ontario. May 30, 1998.

Ruffin, J., Carter, D., Johnston, D., and Baylin, G. "Gluten-free diet for nontropical sprue." *JAMA.* 1964 April 6: 162–4.

Sandison, A. *Degenerative Vascular Diseases in Antiquity.* Brothwell & Sandison (eds.). Springfield, Ill.: Thomas, 1967: 478.

Singh, M., and Kay, S. "Wheat gluten as a pathogenic factor in schizophrenia." *Science.* 1976; 191: 401–2.

Stefansson, V. *Cancer: Disease of Civilization?*, New York: Hill & Wang, 1960, 26.

Swinson, C., Coles, E., Slavin, G., and Booth, C. "Coeliac disease and malignancy." *Lancet.* 1983; 1(8316): 111–5.

Tanchou, S. "Statistics of Cancer." *Lancet.* 1843; Aug 5: 593–4.

Van Berge-Henegouwen, Mulder, C. J. J. "Pioneer in the gluten free diet: Willem-

Karel Dicke 1905–1962, over 50 years of gluten free diet." *Gut.* 1993; 34: 1473–5.

Ventura, A., Magazzu, G., and Greco, L. "Duration of exposure to gluten and risk for autoimmune disorders in patients with celiac disease." *Gastroenterology.* 1999; 117: 297–303.

Wallace, A., and Dohan, F. Curtis. "Medical Researcher." *Philadelphia Inquirer.* Thursday, November 14, 1991.

Zioudrou, C., Streaty, R., and Klee, W. "Opioid peptides derived from food proteins." *J Biol. Chem.* 1979; 254: 2446–9.

Background Sources

Carter, K., and Carter, B. *Childbed Fever.* Westport, Conn.: Greenwood Press, 1994.

Cohen, M. N. "The significance of long-term changes in human diet and food economy," in Harris, M., and Ross, E. (eds). *Food and Evolution: Toward a Theory of Human Food Habits.* Philadelphia: Temple University Press 1987, 261–88.

Embry, A. F., Snowdon, L. R., and Vieth, R. "Vitamin D and seasonal fluctuations of gadolinium-enhancing magnetic resonance imaging lesions in multiple sclerosis." *Ann Neurol.* 2000 Aug; 48(2): 271–2.

Grmek, Mirko D. *Diseases in the Ancient Greek World,* trans. Muellner & Muellner. Baltimore: Johns Hopkins University Press, 1989.

Sigerist, Henry E. *Civilization and Disease.* Chicago: Phoenix Books, University of Chicago Press, 1965 (credits de Latour and Pasteur with much of the germ theory, completely ignoring Semmelweiss's huge contribution).

INDEX